Heart Therapy

Regaining Your
Cardiac Health

Anita Maximin, Psy.D.

Lori Stevic-Rust, Ph.D.

Lori White Kenyon, Ph.D.

New Harbinger Publications, Inc.

Distributed in the U.S.A. by Publishers Group West; in Canada by Raincoast Books; in Great Britain by Airlift Book Company, Ltd.; in South Africa by Real Books, Ltd.; in Australia by Boobook; and in New Zealand by Tandem Press.

Copyright © 1997 by Anita Maximin, Psy.D., Lori Stevic-Rust, Ph.D., and Lori White Kenyon, Ph.D
New Harbinger Publications, Inc.
5674 Shattuck Avenue
Oakland, CA 94609

Cover design by Blue Design, San Francisco, CA.
Text design by Tracy Marie Powell.
Art on pages 27, 29, 109, 111, 124 and 125 by SHELBY DESIGNS & ILLUSTRATES.

Library of Congress Catalog Card Number: 97-75473.
ISBN 1-57224-104-7 Paperback.

New Harbinger Publications' Web address www.newharbinger.com

First printing.

To our parents, who shared the first
and best hearts we have known.

And to all of the patients who have shared
their struggles and battles against heart disease.
May you continue to be strong in heart and spirit.

Contents

There are many people we would like to recognize for their valuable assistance with this project. A treatment manual such as this would not be possible without the valuable contributions of researchers who have devoted their careers to studying cardiac health and prevention of coronary heart disease.

We would like to thank Jim Edmonds for his illustrations, Christine Mitchell for her skilled direction in finding source materials, and Drs. T. J. and R. Maximin for their input on the medical information presented in this book.

We are especially grateful to Rudi Kobetic for readily responding to frantic pleas for computer support.

Thanks to the wonderful staff at New Harbinger: Kristin Beck, for her warmth and exuberance in helping us get this book started; Matt McKay, Lauren Dockett, Gayle Zanca, Kirk Johnson, and the other staff, for their genuine enthusiasm and warm support in all aspects of this project. A special thanks goes to our terrific editor, Farrin Jacobs, for her skillful and meticulous eye for detail and for presenting her feedback in such a gentle manner. Once again, working with New Harbinger has been a pleasurable experience.

Finally, thanks with love, to Skip, Lindsay, and Alex Kenyon; Jay, Sarah, and Katelyn Rust; and Rudi, Vijay, and Ravi Kobetic, who have accepted our juggling of many responsibilities with patience, understanding, and kind support.

Introduction

If you are one of the millions of people who suffers from heart disease, or if you are close to someone who does, you are not alone. More than one in four people have some form of cardiovascular disease. It is the number one killer in our society, more than cancer and all other illnesses combined (American Heart Association 1995). Contrary to the popular perception that heart disease mostly affects middle-aged men, about half of those who die each year are women. In addition, the economic cost is monumental, with about $129 billion in direct health expenses and approximately $21 billion in indirect costs such as lost work time. Therefore, finding ways to reduce the impact of this illness has been a goal for decades. Research has focused on various aspects of heart disease, ranging from finding better treatments that improve and prolong life to prevention of heart diseases.

Researchers have been successful in identifying several risk factors in the development of coronary heart disease. We have divided these risk factors into what we call *traditional risk factors* and *nontraditional risk factors*. Traditional risk factors include high cholesterol, obesity, sedentary lifestyle, smoking, hypertension or high blood pressure, diabetes, and family history. You may be familiar with these risk factors because medical research has primarily focused on them. In addition, organizations such as the National Cholesterol Education Panel and the American Heart Association have instituted programs aimed at increasing public awareness. Your own physicians may have discussed with you only these traditional risk factors.

What may not be as well known to you are what we term non-traditional risk factors, or those related to your emotions. The most commonly talked about emotional risk factor is stress. Experiencing too much stress, as you know, can wear the body down. If you've had a heart attack or suffer from symptoms of heart disease, it may be hard to believe that your emotions could have such a significant connection. Yet factors such as depression, social isolation, your personality style, and stress have been linked with increased risk of heart attacks and poorer recovery after suffering a heart attack. Consider the following statistics: in 1993, Nancy Frasure-Smith and her colleagues found that those who were depressed for a significant period of time after a heart attack had a five to six times greater chance of having another fatal heart attack than those who were not depressed. It is estimated that at least 20 to 40 percent of patients who have suffered a heart attack also suffer from depression. Social isolation—being alone without good support from family or friends—has also been associated with poorer recovery and increased risk of having another heart attack.

Another emotional risk factor that has been studied extensively and linked with heart disease is personality style—that is, the pattern or style in which you relate to your environment and to others. Meyer Friedman, Ray Rosenman, and Diane Ulner (1974, 1984) have looked at what type of personality styles seem to be more coronary-prone. Some of the styles of interacting that have been identified may be a little more difficult for you to admit to having, like an angry, hostile approach to the world or always being impatient or in a hurry. Understandably, these are not traits most people will readily acknowledge in themselves. However, many people who suffer from heart disease possess some of these traits.

We have written this book with the strong belief that your mind and body are connected in ways that are still not well understood. However, based on what is known already, we've found that there are many things you can do to take care of yourself emotionally in order to improve your recovery after a heart attack and decrease your chances of suffering another one. In addition, the traditional risk factors of high cholesterol, smoking, and so on can all be changed by your own choices and actions. The better you manage your stress and other emotions like anger and depression, the less you will be tempted to engage in unhealthy coping behaviors like smoking and not eating well.

Heart Therapy presents a comprehensive approach to keeping your heart healthy. It primarily focuses on coronary heart disease, which is the most preventable of all heart diseases. It is written in an interactive format so that you may actively participate in your own recovery. The book is divided into four parts. Part 1 will give you the necessary basic information about heart disease. Part 2 focuses on your personal adjustment, as well as your family's, to this devastating event. Parts 3 and 4 concentrate on the lifestyle changes you must make in order to have a healthy heart. Part 3 focuses on what you can do to manage traditional risk factors such as your diet, smoking, and getting exercise. Because the lifestyle changes needed to maintain a healthy heart will require motivation and commitment from you, we have included a chapter on the kinds of things that keep people motivated, especially to change longstanding habits and patterns. In part 4, we discuss the most important emotional factors that have been linked with heart disease and give you methods to determine your emotional status, your personality style, and your ability to manage stress. Most importantly, we present some tools to go about changing these aspects if you should need to. Part 5 outlines the special needs of women who have coronary heart disease. Because it was believed in the past that heart disease mostly affected middle-aged men, women were ignored in the research. This has slowly changed in recent years, and particular emphasis has been placed on how women experience heart disease differently from men.

If you have suffered a heart attack, are trying to prevent one, or are close to someone who has, this book is appropriate for you. The evidence is compelling for changing your unhealthy lifestyle habits and unhealthy emotional patterns. Dr. Dean Ornish, in his New York Times best-seller, *Dr. Dean Ornish's Program for Reversing Heart Disease* (1990), writes about the dramatic results of his cardiac recovery program: The participants, all of whom had serious heart disease, participated in a comprehensive program of changing their diet to a lowfat, low-cholesterol one, exercising (in the form of walking and yoga), and learning to manage their stress and feel more connected to others and with themselves. The medical scans of their arteries after a few months of these changes actually showed *reversal* of heart disease, that is, blockages of arteries decreased. They also felt better and required fewer medications. The results of the patients in Dr. Ornish's program, and many others who have been successful in reducing their risk of heart disease by addressing *all* aspects of their lives, offer hope that the same is possible for you. Good luck in your journey to regaining your heart health.

PART 1

Educating Yourself about the Medical Aspects of Heart Disease

Descriptions of the human heart usually fall into one of two camps: the poetic (the heart is the seat of love and compassion) and the scientific (the heart is a highly efficient pumping mechanism). According to the latest research, both views are correct.

—S. Margolis

1

Understanding Your Cardiac Disease: Basic Medical Information

If you have suffered a heart attack or have some other form of cardiac disease, you may be overwhelmed by the amount of information that is presented to you by your physician. Although your doctor may have explained what is happening to your heart, it is difficult to remember everything that was said or to even picture what has happened. This can exacerbate feelings of confusion and anxiety as you try to cope with your illness. You may also have to make some decisions with the help of your cardiologist about what type of treatment you will receive. Therefore, it is important to educate yourself about how the heart works and the type of heart disease that you have.

Anatomy of the Heart Made Simple

The basic function of the heart is to pump oxygenated blood to all the tissues of the body. Oxygen is necessary for our bodies to function. The heart is made up of two upper and two lower *chambers* called the *left atrium, left ventricle, right atrium*, and *right ventricle*. The *right* upper and lower chambers receive the blood from all parts of the body after oxygen has been taken out and then pump that blood to the lungs where the blood is made oxygen-rich again. The oxygen-rich blood then returns to the *left* side of the heart, which, in turn, pumps it out to the various parts of the body. The right chambers are separated from the left chambers by a wall of tissue. The contraction, or the pumping action, of the chambers is coordinated, and the blood flow from the upper chambers to the lower chambers normally occurs only in one direction. Four *valves* act like one-way doors and regulate the flow from one chamber of the heart to another. These are called the *mitral*, the *aortic*, the *tricuspid*, and the *pulmonary* valves. Your "heartbeat" is the pumping action of the heart.

Blood is carried throughout the body by three types of blood vessels: *arteries*, *veins*, and *capillaries*. Arteries carry blood full of oxygen away from the heart. Veins return blood that has been depleted of oxygen by the body back to the heart. Finally, capillaries are very small blood vessels that surround and nourish the tissues. The heart muscle gets its own supply of oxygen-rich blood through special arteries called *coronary arteries*. When these arteries are narrowed by disease, the blood flow to the heart may be markedly decreased and may result in heart attacks.

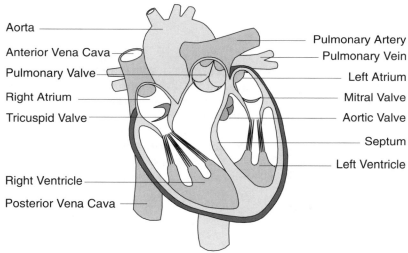

Figure 1.1   The Heart

Types of Cardiac Disease

The heart can have several types of problems with the way it functions. The major types are briefly mentioned here, but the primary focus of this book will be on the most common disease: coronary artery disease.

Atherosclerosis. This is a condition where fatty deposits build up and stick to the walls of arteries, resulting in narrowing of the arteries. This narrowing causes strain on the heart because it has to pump harder. Factors that contribute to the development of atherosclerosis are high cholesterol, high-fat diet, obesity, high blood pressure, diabetes, and smoking. Arteries may become clogged without noticeable symptoms until blood flow is restricted enough to cause chest pain, a heart attack, or a stroke. Because this condition is life-threatening, it's important to prevent or slow down the progress of this disease through lifestyle changes such as healthy eating, exercise, and quitting smoking.

Coronary heart disease (CHD), also referred to as coronary artery disease (CAD). This condition occurs when the blood vessels to the heart (hence the term *coronary artery*) become clogged, thereby making it difficult for blood to flow smoothly to the heart. When the flow of blood is restricted, the heart does not receive the oxygen that it needs to function well. A person can have coronary artery disease without symptoms until the blockage becomes significant enough to cause chest pain. Healthy lifestyle changes can manage CAD.

Angina. Angina is a term for chest pain that results from coronary artery disease. This chest pain occurs when doing stressful activities put strain on a heart that already has to pump harder to get oxygen. Angina can occur frequently and is not an actual heart attack. Simply resting usually alleviates the pain. It is important to have your heart examined carefully if you experience chest pain when exerting yourself or if you have frequent chest pain. Angina could be a warning sign of serious damage to the heart. Treatment options for angina include medications, healthy diet, moderate exercise, and stress reduction. If diagnostic tests show the damage to be severe, then a surgical procedure may be recommended.

Acute myocardial infarction (AMI). A myocardial infarction is the medical term for *heart attack*. A heart attack occurs when the blood flow to a part of the heart muscle is blocked by a blood clot because of a narrowed artery (due to fatty deposits). The part of the heart that is deprived of oxygen becomes damaged. This is different from a *cardiac arrest* where the heart stops beating completely. When the heart stops beating, blood flow to the rest of the body, particularly the brain, also stops, thereby causing death. Brain damage can begin within a few minutes. This is a medical emergency and emergency assistance should be called.

Silent ischemia. With this condition, oxygen supply to the heart cannot keep up with the oxygen demands of the heart because of narrowed arteries. It is a sign of coronary artery disease.

Arrhythmias. An arrhythmia is an irregular heartbeat. Recall that the heartbeat is actually the pumping action of the heart that moves blood throughout the body. *Tachycardia* refers to a rapid heartbeat, which you may experience as a racing heart and intense anxiety. *Atrial fibrillation* occurs when the atrial chambers of the heart do not contract properly and therefore do not empty blood efficiently. The decreased blood flow results in feeling light-headed. *Ventricular fibrillation* is an emergency because the inefficient contractions of the ventricle chambers stop pumping the blood out to the body. Causes of arrhythmias include coronary artery disease and cocaine and alcohol use. If you experience skipped heartbeats, heart palpitations, or unexplained fainting spells, consult with a physician.

Heart valve disease. This involves disease of one or more of the four valves of the heart, with problems with the mitral and aortic valve occurring the most. Disease occurs as a result of deterioration with age, congenital (born with it) abnormalities, or rheumatic fever. The problem can be either narrowing of the valve or leaking of blood backwards (remember, valves are like one-way doors).

Congestive heart failure. This is a condition where the heart has difficulty pumping due to a variety of problems and, therefore, it is not fully effective in maintaining circulation. Symptoms include shortness of breath upon exertion, leg swelling, and accumulation of fluid in the body. One of the causes of congestive heart failure can be muscle damage to the heart from a heart attack.

The functioning of the heart can have multiple problems. The primary focus of this book is on coronary heart disease, which is the one heart disease that can be modified through lifestyle changes. If there are terms and conditions you do not understand or are not covered in this chapter, please ask your physician for an explanation.

2

Signs and Symptoms
of a Heart Attack

Have you ever had pain in your chest or arm that led you to question, "Am I having a heart attack?" You may think it can't happen to you, but about 1.5 million people per year in the United States have heart attacks (also known as *myocardial infarction* or *coronary thrombosis*). Heart attacks are the most common cause of deaths from heart disease in the United States. And not all heart attacks are signaled by the sudden, crushing chest pain often typified on television or in the movies. It's important to familiarize yourself with the range of symptoms that are the early warning signs of a heart attack. Medical treatments for heart attacks have progressed greatly in recent years, which means that your chances of surviving a heart attack and your potential for a good recovery are better than ever. But this is true only if you get appropriate medical attention quickly.

The first hour of a heart attack has been termed *the golden hour*. If you get medical treatment during that first hour, your chances of recovery are vastly improved. Medical treatments such as the clot-busting medications (thrombolytics), which dissolve blockages in coronary arteries and restore blood flow to the heart, are effective only if administered soon after the onset of the attack. Clot-dissolving medications probably are of little benefit if given more than six hours after your symptoms began. Delay in seeking treatment for symptoms of a heart attack can be deadly. So again, learning the range of signs indicating a potential heart attack is critical.

The symptoms associated with a heart attack vary, which can make decisions about seeking help confusing. Sometimes heart attacks can come on gradually over time, preceded by a few weeks of angina.

They can also happen suddenly, without any warning. The main symptom is usually a squeezing pain in the center of your chest. Heart attack victims often describe their pain as one or more of the following: dull, crushing, heavy, constricting, pressurelike, tight, squeezing. The pain may spread to your neck, upper jaw, shoulders, or arms (usually the left arm). However, many heart attacks start with mild symptoms that may not be considered painful. Early symptoms include feeling dizzy, weak, light-headed, or as if you may faint. Some heart attacks are accompanied by great difficulty breathing—feeling like you can't catch your breath—heavy sweating, upset stomach, or vomiting. Doctors now recommend that you get help immediately if you experience any of the following symptoms for more than two minutes, or if you have symptoms that return after going away:

- Chest pain or discomfort (this can range from a crushing pain in the center of your chest to uncomfortable pressure, fullness, or squeezing sensations)

- Pain spreading to your jaw, neck, shoulders, or either arm

- Chest pain or discomfort accompanied by dizziness, light-headedness, sudden weakness, or fainting

- Chest pain or discomfort accompanied by sweating, chills, shortness of breath, nausea or vomiting

- Angina episodes where your symptoms do not get better after taking medication (nitroglycerin), or episodes of angina that come much more frequently, last longer, or are much more intense than in the past

Whether you are male or female, you may experience any combination of these symptoms during a heart attack. Men having heart attacks are somewhat more likely than women to have the crushing or squeezing chest pain as a symptom. Women are somewhat more likely to have symptoms including shortness of breath, fatigue, chest discomfort or pressure rather than pain, or pain from the jaw to the diaphragm.

You may be more likely to have a heart attack at certain times of the day or under certain circumstances. In general, heart attacks seem more easily triggered at the following times:

- *Soon after awakening.* You're about twice as likely to have a heart attack within two hours after awakening than at other times of the day. It may be to your benefit, especially if you have heart disease or risk factors for it, to get out of bed slowly and take a relaxed pace in the mornings. It may also be advisable to avoid physically or emotionally strenuous tasks soon after arising from bed.

- *During or immediately after periods of heavy physical activity or exertion.* You may be almost six times more likely to have a heart attack within one hour of heavy exertion as compared to less strenuous or no activity levels. This relationship has been shown only in men, probably because women, especially of advancing ages, are less likely to engage in physically strenuous activities. But this doesn't mean that this isn't a risk for women as well. You can protect yourself from this risk by physically conditioning your heart and your body. Engaging in regular exercise can strengthen your heart so it does not become as strained during activities requiring more exertion.

- *During or closely after periods of emotional distress.* Emotional upset appears to be the most common triggering factor for heart attacks. Studies have found that roughly 20 percent of heart attack victims say that they experienced emotional stress—either positive or negative—in the two hours before their heart attack symptoms began (Allan and Scheidt 1996). For example, the shock of hearing of a death of a loved one appears to increase your risk of a heart attack by about 13 percent.

- *During or closely following episodes of anger.* Within the two hours following an angry outburst, you may be more than twice as likely to have a heart attack than at nonangry times. Mittleman, MacLure, Sherwood, and colleagues (1995) described that the most frequent causes of anger leading to heart attacks include arguments with family, work conflicts, or legal problems. They suggested that if you take aspirin regularly (one aspirin every other day), you may eliminate the risk associated with your body's physical response to anger, which includes a surge in adrenaline, increased heart rate and blood pressure, and changes that make blood more likely to clot. Aspirin may decrease the likelihood of blood clots forming, even during angry times. Learning ways to relax is also helpful in coping with anger and in reducing your body's reactions to these episodes.

Action Steps

A heart attack is a medical emergency. If you or someone you know has the symptoms, immediately call an ambulance or your physician, who may want to meet you at the emergency room. If a telephone is not available, or someone can drive you to the hospital more quickly than waiting for an ambulance, then go to the nearest emergency room that offers twenty-four-hour emergency cardiac care. If you are with someone experiencing signs of a heart attack that last for more than a few minutes, act immediately. The American Heart Association recommends the following action steps:

1. Expect a denial. It's normal for someone with chest discomfort to deny the possibility of something as serious as a heart attack. Do not take "no" for an answer. Act immediately.

2. If the person is unconscious, check to be sure that his or her airway is open and check for breathing and pulse. If you don't detect a pulse, start CPR (mouth-to-mouth breathing with chest compressions) if you are trained in this.

3. If the person is conscious, help him or her to the least painful position (usually half-sitting with legs supported by a pillow under the knees).

4. Loosen any tight clothing and don't allow any unnecessary movements.

5. If the person has nitroglycerin, use it within the guidelines suggested by the doctor.

6. Aspirin helps prevent blood platelets from sticking together and forming a clot or enlarging a clot that already exists. The American Heart Association (Hennekens et al. 1997) suggests that there is clear and conclusive evidence that aspirin is beneficial. Taking aspirin at the onset of chest pain or other symptoms of a heart attack can improve chances for a good recovery. Researchers estimate that up to ten thousand lives per year could be saved with the use of aspirin. A physician should be consulted about whether aspirin therapy is appropriate and what dosage should be taken.

7. Do not give the person anything to eat or drink.

Especially if you have a history of heart disease or are at increased risk due to risk factors, you need to become familiar with the warning signs of a heart attack, as well as what actions to take. The American Heart Association also suggests that you prepare for emergencies in advance by finding out which hospitals in your area offer twenty-four-hour emergency cardiac care. Let your family and friends know of your preferred hospital, and keep emergency numbers handy.

Can Symptoms Be Something Other Than a Heart Attack?

Symptoms of a heart attack might not reflect cardiac difficulties at all but may stem from other conditions. For instance, many of the symptoms mentioned can be brought on by digestive disorders, thyroid problems, muscle strain, or an anxiety disorder. People who suffer from panic attacks often believe they are having a heart attack, because symptoms of an anxiety attack can include one or more of the potential symptoms of a heart attack.

So how do you tell if your symptoms are a heart attack or are something else? The bottom line is, it's better to be safe than sorry. Only an examination by a medical professional, often including various medical tests, can determine for sure if you are having a heart attack. Especially if this is the first time you have had these symptoms, don't wait to see if you feel better: immediate medical attention is necessary. There is no need to feel embarrassed if your symptoms turn out to be anxiety, or "just gas." The statistics show that only about 15 percent of people who go to the emergency room for symptoms of a heart attack are actually diagnosed with a heart attack (Cunningham et al. 1989; Ting et al. 1991). Emergency room doctors are used to false alarms.

If your symptoms are related to anxiety, you may have a condition called *panic disorder*. This is marked by repeated and unpredictable episodes of anxiety. Symptoms may include

- Racing, pounding heart
- Chest pains
- Light-headedness or dizziness
- Flushes or chills
- Difficulty catching your breath
- Trembling
- Numbness or tingling in arms
- Fear of dying

For the majority of persons with this disorder, symptoms reflect the body's response to anxiety and not heart disease. Most people having panic attacks do not die or have heart attacks, though this is the common fear. A thorough medical exam is necessary to rule out any cardiac or other physical difficulties. If you have been reassured by your doctor that you do not have any heart problems, then you probably do not need to seek medical treatment for your symptoms each time they occur. Instead, you can learn ways of relaxing and controlling anxiety symptoms so you no longer feel compelled to seek emergency medical treatment. Although up to ten million Americans have panic disorder, only about one-third of them get the proper treatment. Psychological counseling techniques and a variety of medications are available and have been shown to be highly effective in treating panic disorder. If you have problems with anxiety, talk with your doctor about treatment options. If left untreated, anxiety can make your life miserable and be harmful to your heart. People who are chronically tense, nervous, and anxious are more likely to have abnormal heart rhythms and are at greater risk of sudden death from heart disease.

Can Heart Attacks Be Silent?

Have you been asked by a doctor about a prior heart attack, when you didn't realize you'd had a prior attack? Sometimes heart attacks occur with few or no symptoms—or at least no symptoms that are associated with a heart attack. This is called *silent infarction*, or *unrecognized infarction*, and is diagnosed by evidence from a medical test, such as an EKG. This is important, of course, because if you don't recognize having symptoms of a heart attack, then you will not seek treatment for it either.

The Framingham Heart Study, which has followed four thousand Massachusetts men for more than forty years, has found that about 25 percent of heart attacks go unnoticed until detected on annual EKGs. As many as a third to half of all heart attacks may be silent (Condos 1996; Anderson 1991). Researchers have tried to identify medical factors that may be related to silent infarction, but results have not been consistent. Some studies suggest that you may be at greater risk of silent heart attack if you are female, of older age, have high blood pressure, diabetes, or if you smoke (Bertolet and Hill 1989). But these findings have not been definitive. Researchers suggest that the more risk factors you have for heart disease, the more likely you may be to have a silent heart attack. For example, if you are a man over age fifty, a diabetic, and a smoker—or a postmenopausal woman, overweight, with high cholesterol levels—then you are likely at increased risk. Dr. William Condos Jr. (1996), Medical Director of the Cardiovascular Institute of the South, suggests that if you have three or more risk factors for heart disease, you should consider asking your physician about a screening for silent ischemia (reduced oxygen in the heart that does not lead to pain). A screening would probably include a medical history questionnaire, physical examination, and cardiac stress (exercise) test.

Do Not Delay in Seeking Treatment for Heart Attack Symptoms

If you've never had a heart attack, it may be hard for you to believe how or why people experiencing heart attack symptoms would hesitate to get help. However, it's common for persons having a heart attack to hesitate to seek treatment—for a variety of reasons. As mentioned earlier, you may not experience any significant symptoms that you associate with heart difficulties, even while you're having a heart attack. Symptoms may be mild or not painful. Additionally, it may be hard for you to accept the possibility of a serious illness like heart attack.

About half of all heart attack victims wait more than two hours before getting help. A substantial number wait more than twelve hours! This kind of delay limits your chances of survival, because most heart attack victims who die do so within a few minutes to two hours of the onset of symptoms. The majority of these sudden cardiac deaths appear related to abnormal patterns of heart rate (arrhythmias) that could often be reversed with prompt medical attention.

The importance of time cannot be emphasized strongly enough. When a coronary artery gets blocked, the heart muscle does not die instantly, but damage increases the longer the artery is blocked. If a victim gets to the emergency room quickly enough, then a form of therapy that dissolves the blockage (thrombolytic medications) may be performed. These medications must be given within several hours of the onset of the heart attack for you to receive the greatest benefits. Early treatment with these drugs has been associated with lower mortality rates, smaller areas of heart muscle damage, and improved heart functioning after the heart attack. These drugs cannot be given to everyone because they have side effects (such as possible bleeding in various organs) that may lead doctors to avoid using them in some cases. However, avoiding delay is still important: many other forms of therapy can also be life-saving.

Delay in beginning treatment can be related to

- The time it takes you to decide to seek help

- The time needed for transportation to the hospital

- The time taken in the hospital to diagnose a heart attack and begin treatment for it

In most cases, the time it takes people to decide to get help is the longest part of the total delay time. Whether you are male or female, older or younger, or of a particular race does not seem to consistently affect how long you will wait. Surprisingly, even having had a prior heart attack does not appear to lead people to get help more quickly for a subsequent attack.

Several studies have indicated that your emotions and personality traits may influence how long you wait before seeking treatment for symptoms of a heart attack (Matthews et al. 1983; Freedland et al. 1991; Kenyon et al. 1991). You may be at risk of lengthy delays if you are a pressured, easily aggravated, Type A personality. In addition, you may delay longer if you're not very aware of your inner bodily and emotional signals. People range from those who are sensitive and alert to signals from their bodies, including emotional states, to those who don't easily identify or acknowledge what's happening on the inside—both in terms of physical signs and emotions. This tendency to avoid or lack contact with inner feelings has been labeled *alexithymia*, which is a Greek word meaning "no words for emotions." Both Type A persons and those who are alexithymic tend to focus outwardly on activities instead of inwardly on what's happening inside of their bodies. If you have one of these styles of responding, you may tend to ignore or postpone attention to distress signals from your body. Or you may react to internal signals of distress by immediately throwing yourself into some activity, which allows you to put the pain out of your mind. For example, many heart attack victims will engage in a number of actions in attempts to ward off their symptoms. Activities like taking antacids, painkillers, or trying to walk off or sleep off the pain are not unusual.

A group of researchers from Detroit, Michigan, recently found that heart attack victims who were unaware of emotional or physical signals in themselves were likely to delay much longer than those showing better awareness of emotions and physical senses (Kenyon et al. 1991). Those persons out of touch emotionally and physically tended to wait so long that treatment options were usually limited. People more aware of feelings and physical signs arrived at the emergency room, on the average, in four hours or less—the time frame allowing for a greater range of treatment options and increasing chances for a better outcome.

You can tell if you are out of touch with emotional and physical signals from your body by answering the following questions:

1. Is it hard for you to put your feelings into words? Do you usually use general descriptors, like "good," "bad," "it hurts," "it feels good"? _____

2. Do others ask you to describe your feelings more? _____

3. Do you tend to focus almost always on the tasks at hand and rarely, if ever, daydream? _____

4. Do you feel daydreaming is a waste of time? _____

5. Do you believe that it's not important to be in touch with feelings? _____

6. Is it hard for you to understand emotions in others close to you? _____

7. Are you rarely troubled by bodily aches and pains? _____

If you responded "yes" to at least half of these questions, then you may have a tendency to ignore emotions and physical sensations. Don't despair. You can train yourself to pay more attention to internal signals and feelings. This is particularly important if you have already had a heart attack and you delayed excessively—more than two hours—in getting treatment.

Try these techniques to enhance your inner focus:

- Learn, and frequently refresh your familiarity with, the range of warning signs of a heart attack.

- Take time daily (twenty minutes may be enough) to sit or lie in a soothing position and focus on relaxing the muscles in your body.

- When you notice a fleeting physical sensation in your body, don't gloss over it. Stop and assess it. Talk with your physician about what natural bodily responses are and which signal problems related to your heart.

- When you feel "upset" or "good," take time to consider your feelings more carefully and try to be more specific in labeling them. Are you angry, sad, lonely, insecure? Are you happy, proud, joyful, relieved, loving? Consider factors that have led you to feel this way. By doing this, you can better deal with and express your feelings instead of glossing over them and focusing too much on the tasks at hand.

- Learn that feelings are not silly or meaningless and should not be habitually ignored. Instead, they signal important information that—if you can reflect upon it—can help you respond better to stressful events and to life in general.

3

What Can Be Done:
Medical Procedures
and Treatment

How a Diagnosis Is Made

Several tests, ranging from simple to more invasive, are used to diagnose cardiac disease. When you experience symptoms that may indicate a heart attack, your doctor will send you for further testing to determine the nature of the problem. Educating yourself about the different diagnostic tests will help alleviate some of your anxiety. The following is a general description of some of the tests and what they help to determine.

Electrocardiogram (EKG or ECG)

This is usually the first test that your doctor may order for you. It measures the patterns of electrical activity in the heart. It is the electrical impulses from the cells of the heart that contract the heart muscles in a regular rhythm, which, in turn, pump the blood throughout the body. An EKG can measure abnormalities in the heart's rhythm; it will indicate whether there has been a previous heart attack, an enlarged heart, or other signs that may indicate problems with your heart.

During an EKG, the patient is asked to lie down, and electrodes, or *leads*, are placed on his or her chest. The leads are then connected to a machine called an *electrocardiograph* that records the electrical impulses of the heart. The pattern of the electrical activity is recorded on a long, narrow strip of paper and then examined for abnormal spikes and patterns. This test usually takes about fifteen minutes.

Stress EKG, or Exercise Tolerance Test

This test, also known as the *treadmill test*, is basically an EKG done while exercising on a treadmill or a stationary bicycle. The stress EKG can detect the presence of severe heart disease on most occasions and can also fairly accurately detect coronary artery disease. As in the plain EKG, electrodes are placed on different parts of the patient's chest. The patient then begins walking on a treadmill or riding a bike. Blood pressure, heart rate, and the EKG patterns are monitored as the pace of the exercise increases. The pace may increase to a level much more than what the patient is normally accustomed to. The whole test takes about thirty minutes.

This test is very important to take before you start on a strenuous exercise program if you are over forty years old and/or if you have (or your family has) a history of heart disease, high blood pressure, high cholesterol, or if you are a smoker. If the test results show that you have some heart disease, your doctor will establish safe guidelines for your exercise.

Holter Monitoring

The Holter monitor is a small device connected to one or two leads of the EKG that the patient wears for a twenty-four-hour period. The patient is requested to go about the activities of a typical day while keeping notes of any symptoms. Symptoms that are noted by the patient can then be compared to the EKG to see whether or not there are any problems with how the heart is working and during what type of activities. The Holter monitor is most useful for evaluating heart arrhythmias and silent ischemia.

Echocardiography

Also known as *cardiac ultrasonography*, this test uses the sound waves bouncing from the heart to create a pattern that is then amplified as three-dimensional images on a screen. Echocardiogram findings are also recorded on graph paper. This test can provide information about the heart's pumping action, its size, structures, and patterns. It can help diagnose conditions such as damage from a heart attack, narrowing of the aorta, fluid in the sac around the heart, heart valve problems, heart muscle disease, and cardiac tumors.

The procedure for an echocardiogram is similar to that of an ultrasound. A cardiologist, radiologist, or ultrasound technician places a device called a transducer on the patient's chest. The sound waves are reflected back onto a screen that shows the structure and activity of the heart.

Radionuclide Scans

This type of test is also called a *thallium exercise scan*. Thallium, a radioactive substance, is injected in a very small amount into the arm while the patient is on a treadmill. A "picture" of the heart is then obtained in which dark areas on the scan indicate where blood flow is impaired. A thallium exercise scan is typically the next step if there is an abnormal EKG finding. It is important to follow through because an abnormal EKG finding may mean that your heart is not working properly.

Cardiac Catheterization

This procedure is used to determine the amount of blockage or narrowing of the coronary arteries. The test is done in a specially equipped laboratory in the hospital. In this procedure, a flexible tube, called a *catheter*, is inserted into an artery either in the groin area or in the upper arm and slowly guided up through the artery to the heart and to the coronary arteries. A dye that is injected into the catheter flows through the bloodstream, allowing X rays of the heart and its arteries to be taken. This type of X ray is called an *angiogram*. There are some risks associated with this procedure, such as unexpected reaction to the dye, irregular and rapid heart rhythm, or even cardiac arrest. These events are not common, however, and should they occur, they can be managed by your cardiologist and the staff in the specialized laboratory.

Ultrafast CT Scans

This new technique has evolved over the past three years or so and holds promise in providing further information about the risks of heart disease. The procedure is a refinement of what you know as CT scans, or *computed tomographic scans*. CT scans are commonly used procedures that provide clear views of many internal body structures. As recently discussed in the *Johns Hopkins Medical Letter: Health After 50* (June 1997), ultrafast CT scanning is a "sped-up" CT scan that allows evaluation of coronary arteries even though they are in constant motion.

The scan provides information about how much calcium is in your arteries. It's not exactly known why calcium collects in your arteries (it appears unrelated to the amount of calcium you eat), but once there, it appears to contribute to atherosclerosis (hardening and narrowing of the arteries). Research suggests that levels of calcium in your arteries may be a better predictor of heart disease than cholesterol, blood pressure, smoking, or family history of heart disease. This technique may allow physicians to detect signs of heart disease earlier than the commonly used stress test. This is especially important for those people who do not notice any symptoms that signal their heart disease, as is the case in silent heart attack or silent ischemia (a drop in blood flow to the heart that is not accompanied by any symptoms).

A recent study by Budhoff et al., reported in the cardiology journal *Circulation* (1996), indicated that results of ultrafast CT scans were about ten times better than cholesterol level tests at predicting who would have problems with heart disease. This technique has not yet become a routine procedure used in diagnosing heart disease. However, the American Heart Association believes that the method is a promising way to gauge risks in people who may not have symptoms of heart disease but who have risk factors for it. This way, treatments could be initiated earlier, possibly leading to better outcomes.

Coping with Anxiety about Potential Results

Although the results you receive may be serious, it will be important to not let your anxiety interfere with hearing what your doctor is telling you. If you have had a heart attack or been diagnosed with coronary artery disease or another type of cardiac illness, you will face some decisions about what type of intervention you may need. Denying that the problem exists because of fear of further medical procedures or fear about what the results mean for your life will only be potentially dangerous to your health. Your cardiologist will inform you about your condition, risks to your health, and available treatments. By receiving this information as early as possible and beginning any recommended treatments, you will minimize your chances of suffering from another cardiac event.

Getting the Most out of Your Health Care

Before you go to your doctor's office to hear the review of your test results, it will be helpful to prepare yourself in advance. Here are some suggestions that may assist you in getting the most out of your office visit and reducing your anxiety

Become an active participant in your health care. This will increase some sense of control over your life at a time when everything that is happening to you feels as though it's beyond your control.

Write down a list of questions and concerns that you have. It's difficult to remember everything that you might like to ask your doctor when you're in the midst of hearing life-altering news. It may be helpful to take a notepad with you and ask the doctor to make a sketch of the medical procedure and diagram of the damage or blockages to your arteries and heart muscle. Sometimes it's easier to understand what is happening when you can envision it. In addition, it may be helpful to take the following list with you to remind you of important questions to ask:

- Could you describe my medical condition in specific terms?
- What did my test results reveal?
- What are the expectations for recovery?
- What are my risk factors?
- Could you describe all of the potential interventions?
- What kind of symptoms should be reported immediately?
- Which hospital should I go to in case of emergency?
- What activities am I restricted from and for how long?

Write down the information that the doctor gives you in your notepad for later review. You will be hearing a lot of new and potentially anxiety-provoking information. It will be helpful to write this information down so that you can discuss it with your family, read further about your condition, or just simply absorb all of it at a slower pace.

Remember that you will not have to make any decisions immediately. With the exception of an emergency, you will have some time to adjust to your diagnosis before you have any further interventions. But keep in mind, early detection and intervention are essential for reducing your risk for additional cardiac problems.

Consider taking a family member or friend with you to your appointment. Your spouse, partner, family, and/or friends can give you the support you'll need at this time. Your spouse or partner in particular will be most closely involved with your care. Including them at your appointment will not only help alleviate some of their concerns, but they may also think of questions that you have not or that you might forget to ask.

Types of Treatment

Generally, the major treatment categories for coronary heart disease are *interventional* and *pharmacological (drug) therapy*. The third major treatment for heart disease involves lifestyle changes. Information about such changes forms the bulk of this cardiac health book and is discussed in subsequent chapters. You will most likely use a combination of all three types for the treatment of your heart disease. In fact, the success of the medical interventions and the drug therapy will be improved if you can make the necessary lifestyle changes as well.

There are other heart conditions that are not as readily modifiable through lifestyle changes as coronary heart disease. These conditions include inflammation of the lining of the heart, malfunction of the valves of the heart, and disturbances in the rhythm of the heart. These are often treated with medications, open-heart surgery, and in extreme cases, heart transplant.

Medical Intervention

The most traditional forms of treatment for coronary heart disease are medical procedures that aim to open up narrowed blood vessels and medications that control factors such as high blood pressure and cholesterol levels. The following is a description of each of these procedures.

Angioplasty

The full medical term for this procedure is *percutaneous transluminal coronary angioplasty* (PCTA). The procedure is similar to that of the cardiac catheterization: a small deflated balloon attached to the end of a catheter is inserted into the femoral artery in the groin area. It is then passed all the way up through the aorta to the blood vessel in the heart that is blocked by fatty plaques. Plaques are caused by the accumulation of cholesterol and other substances, such as platelets, on the walls of arteries, resulting in thickening of the vessel wall and subsequent narrowing or blockage of that blood vessel. The blockage must be partial so that there is space to maneuver the deflated balloon. The balloon is then inflated in a controlled manner (it cannot exceed a certain size) so that the plaques become squashed out of the way, thereby allowing the blood to flow more freely. The inflation period lasts for about thirty to ninety seconds, and it may be necessary to do it more than one time. The blood vessels that are amenable to this procedure are chosen based on location and whether there is a low risk of potential damage. Patients can usually be back to doing regular activities within two or three days.

Cardiologists are careful not to stretch or tear the wall of the artery, but sometimes this complication can occur. Usually it causes no significant problems, and the patient is given medication to control the clotting system of the blood for a period of time. The most common problem with angioplasty is the return of the plaques within three to six months; this occurs in about 30 to 35 percent of patients. Patients who have regrowth of the fatty deposits after a couple angioplasties may need surgery.

Other types of angioplasty work similarly to the standard balloon angioplasty. They include using laser surgery to destroy the plaques or devices that cut away some of the plaques (*atherectomy*). Their success rate is similar to that of standard balloon angioplasty. *Stents* are tiny metal devices that are inserted through a catheter to support the vessel wall and prevent growth of further plaques. Stents help keep the angioplasty site open.

Before you have a procedure such as balloon angioplasty, ask your cardiologist about his or her experience in performing this procedure. A recent study (Ellis et al. 1997) provides evidence suggesting that the more experience doctors have with performing this procedure, the lower the complication rates tend to be. For example, the rate of complications for doctors who had done more than 270 such procedures in the prior year was less than 3 percent, whereas it was over 9 percent for those doctors who had performed fewer than 70 angioplasties in the prior year.

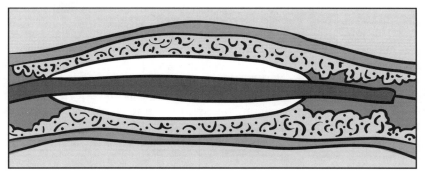

Figure 2.1   Balloon Angioplasty

Coronary Artery Bypass Graft (CABG)

This surgery is used to treat a clogged or blocked coronary artery. The heart is accessed by opening up the body through the breastbone. The blocked artery is *bypassed*, or *grafted*, with another healthy artery, which then provides a clear passageway for blood to reach the heart. The new passageway to the heart is attached to the aorta and then to the blocked artery at a position downstream from the blockage. The new blood vessel is usually one of the arteries that run alongside the breastbone (called the left internal mammary artery, or LIMA) or a portion of a vein from the upper or lower leg (saphenous vein grafts, or SVGs). Such new grafts come from areas of the body where there are extra blood vessels to supply that part of the body. Depending on the number of arteries that are bypassed the procedure is referred to as a double, triple, or quadruple bypass, or a CABG times two, three, or four, respectively.

The CABG (often pronounced by health professionals as "cabbage") surgery takes about four hours, depending on how many arteries need to be bypassed. During the surgery, the heart is stopped and emptied of blood. A heart-lung machine (cardiopulmonary bypass) takes over pumping blood through the body. The success rate is over 90 percent in stopping chest pain for at least five to ten years after the surgery. The major reason why this surgery is so successful is that, for some unknown reason, most people develop the fatty plaques only in certain segments of their arteries, not throughout the entire artery. Some segments of an artery may be partially or completely blocked while a little farther down, the artery is completely clean. Therefore, bypassing the diseased area seems to be the simplest and most effective way around the problem. Approximately 350,000 CABG surgeries are performed every year in the United States.

New techniques are being developed as alternatives to the traditional CABG operations. Doctors at Johns Hopkins Medical Center and the Cleveland Clinic are perfecting a technique called *minimally invasive bypass*, or *buttonhole* or *keyhole* bypass. The advantage of these procedures is that instead of major surgery opening the breastbone and ribcage—as required for CABG surgeries—small buttonhole incisions are made in the chest. The surgeons then insert miniature scopes and scalpels through these holes and perform the bypass operation using a view of the heart they see projected on a TV screen in the operating room. Because this procedure is so new, it's not yet certain how success rates compare with the traditional bypass operation (CABG). If you are considering a traditional bypass operation, ask your doctor about possible alternatives such as a less invasive approach.

Drug Therapy

The other major form of treatment you are likely to receive is drug therapy. In order to reduce your risk of having another heart attack, many medications have been developed to help control various factors such as blood pressure, heart rate, and the way your blood clots. If you've been diagnosed with heart disease of any type, including coronary artery disease, you should expect to take medications on a daily basis. Some of these medications may have side effects, but usually the benefit of reducing your risk of another heart attack far outweighs the side effects. It is likely that you may be prescribed more than one type of medication. Remembering when and how many to take of each can sometimes be difficult, because some should be taken with food to avoid an upset stomach and others on an empty stomach. A further complication is that many of the medications may resemble each other in size and color.

Try to learn as much as you can about your medications. Begin by asking your doctor the following questions:

- What is each medication for and what results are expected? That is, what is it supposed to do?

- What are the generic or brand names of each medication?

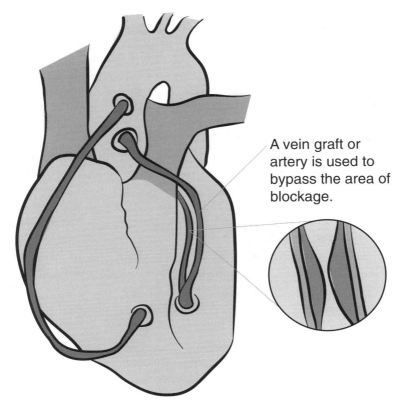

A vein graft or artery is used to bypass the area of blockage.

Figure 2.2   Coronary Artery Bypass Graft

- How much should I take at one time, how often, when? With food or on an empty stomach?
- Do I need to avoid any foods or alcohol while taking these medications?
- What over-the-counter medications or drugs prescribed by any other doctor do I need to be careful about when taking this medication?
- What are possible side effects? What are the treatments for any unpleasant side effects?
- What symptoms should I report immediately? How long should I wait before calling you if I have any problems?
- Will it be safe to drive or operate other heavy machinery?
- Will any of the medications affect my ability to perform at work?
- Are there any psychological side effects, like depression or anxiety?

Writing down the information will be useful for later reference. Your doctor may also have some printed literature on some of the medications that are prescribed for you.

The effectiveness of your medications will depend on you taking them properly. The medication containers may not be labeled with all of the instructions, so keep the information you receive from your doctor handy as a reference. The following tips will assist you in remembering to take your medications appropriately:

- Plan to take your medications at the same time every day so that it becomes routine. It's often helpful to take them either right before or during your meals as advised by your doctor. If you miss a dose by several hours, ask your doctor if you should skip the dosage or go on to the next time. *Do not double up without first consulting your doctor.*

- Making a chart or checklist of medications that you need to take each day can be helpful if you have trouble remembering.

- You may want to color code your medication bottles if you have trouble reading them. Make a note on your chart or checklist of what color you choose to mark each drug.

- Use a pill organizer available at your local drugstore. Pill organizers are little plastic containers divided into compartments; you can get seven-day pill containers that are marked for each day of the week and for morning, noon, and night. You can also get smaller-sized pill containers for travel if you plan on being away for the day. Electronic pill organizers are also available at a local drugstore or electronic store. These can be set with alarms that remind you when it's time to take your medications. Using the alarm on your wristwatch can also be helpful.

- If there are places away from home where you spend time regularly, plan to keep a backup or emergency supply of medications. For instance, you may be prescribed nitroglycerin in case of chest pain or discomfort; you should carry a supply with you at all times and have some in your car, at work, and any other place where you regularly visit.

- Select a pharmacy near you and get to know the pharmacist. Pharmacists can be very helpful in providing you with information about medication dosages, interactions with other medications, side effects, and so on. Make sure that the pharmacist is accessible and willing to answer any questions. Also select a pharmacy or backup pharmacy that is available at night and during weekends.

- Some of the medications prescribed for you will be expensive. Ask your pharmacy about their payment options. Do they accept your prescription insurance plan? Can you pay by credit card? Can you be billed monthly?

- Some of your medications may be available at a discount through mail order if you purchase them in larger quantities or repeatedly over time. The American Association of Retired Persons (AARP) has a list of mail order pharmacy services. Their phone number is (202) 434-2277.

Following is a brief description of each class of medications that are commonly used for the treatment of heart disease.

Beta-Blockers

This group of medications is used to slow your heart rate, lower blood pressure, and decrease the strength of your heart contraction. It is used to treat conditions such as high blood pressure, angina, and arrhythmias. Beta-blockers are also typically prescribed after someone has had a heart attack. Brand names include Inderal, Blocadren, Lopressor, Toprol, Tenormin, Corgard, Sectral, and Visken.

ACE Inhibitors

ACE inhibitors belong to a class of drugs known as vasodilators, which relax blood vessels by acting on the muscle wall of the vessel. ACE stands for *angiotensin converting enzyme*. Angiotensin is an enzyme in your body that causes arteries to constrict. ACE is needed to make angiotensin active. ACE inhibitors block the action of this enzyme and therefore open, or dilate, your blood vessels. These are excellent drugs for the treatment of high blood pressure. They are also used in people who have congestive heart failure. Brand names include Capoten, Lotensin, Vasotec, Monopril, Zestril, Prinivil, Accupril, and Altace.

Calcium Channel Blockers

This class of drugs also relaxes your blood vessels (vasodilators). Therefore, they are used to treat high blood pressure. Brand names include Adalat CC, Cardizem, Dilacor, Procardia, Cardene, Norvasc, Calan, and Isoptin.

Nitrates

Nitrate drugs dilate the blood vessels of the heart and therefore are used to treat chest pain. They are made from nitroglycerin (yes, the same chemical as the explosive). Nitrates are usually taken by placing a pill under your tongue or as a patch on your skin. You may be required to carry some nitroglycerin pills with you at all times in case of emergency, for example, acute chest pain. Brand names include Sorbitrate, Isordil, and Transderm-Nitro.

Diuretics

This group of drugs removes excess fluid and salt from your body by increasing urine output. Some can also dilate your vessels; dilated vessels and less fluid in your body brings down your blood pressure. Brand names include Lasix, Edecrin, and Esidrex.

Anti-lipid Agents

These drugs work in various ways, depending on the drug, to reduce atherosclerosis (fatty plaques) in your blood vessels. Some improve your levels of good cholesterol, or high-density lipoprotein (HDL), and others reduce your total cholesterol and bad cholesterol, low-density lipoprotein (LDL). The most widely used include Mevacor, Zocor, Lescol, and Pravachol.

Anticoagulants

These drugs interfere with clotting of blood, which reduces your chance of having a clot block blood flow in one of the coronary arteries. The most widely used anticoagulant is Coumadin. It is typically given to patients who've had a massive heart attack.

Thrombolytics

Also known as clot-busters, these drugs break up clots that are blocking a blood vessel. They are given immediately after a heart attack to minimize damage to the heart muscle. Examples include tissue plasminogen activator (tPA), streptokinase, and urokinase.

Aspirin

Aspirin has been shown to be effective in protecting against clot formation in coronary arteries and other places in the body. Large-scale studies have shown that aspirin can reduce the risk of recurrent heart attack and possibly help reduce risk of heart attack in those who do not have coronary heart disease. It's important to take the aspirin with meals to prevent stomach upset.

Anxiety Associated with Medical Procedures

Have you ever experienced a crisis of some kind in your life? Perhaps you have had a crisis within your family or with your children. Maybe a divorce, car accident, financial difficulties, illness in the family, and so on. A crisis is the point where a sudden and abrupt change occurs and is seen as a turning point either for the better or worse. A crisis point in a medical illness can be the time when the condition worsens or improves. Usually when people are going through a crisis situation they report feeling out of control, frightened, and worried about their ability to cope with the event. Medical and surgical procedures have been described as crises by several researchers because, like other nonmedical crises in our lives, they can also make us feel out of control and fearful about our ability to cope with the pain and possible consequences of the procedures.

During a crisis situation you can become immobile and temporarily unable to respond in a healthy way. Without healthy and adaptive coping strategies, you will be unable to reduce your anxiety and effectively cope with the crisis. When people are exposed to a crisis situation, they first begin to assess and interpret the harmful nature of the situation as well as their *ability* to deal with the anxiety that it arouses within us. Remember, a crisis situation or event is usually experienced as sudden and abrupt even if it's related to a chronic condition and as such can leave you feeling overwhelmed and at a loss for how to begin to cope. For instance, even if you had warning about your cardiac disease, the need for an invasive medical or surgical procedure probably felt like a new change or stressor to cope with. Perhaps the need for a procedure made your illness suddenly feel real and frightening. You could no longer deny or ignore the seriousness of your condition. The procedure may actually have been the turning point that made you face the reality of your disease.

Maybe you've recently been told that you need a medical procedure or you have already been through one and are fearful of the need for another one in the future. Although it is fairly common to experience anxiety and fear about medical procedures, it is important to manage it because extreme anxiety can interfere with the actual procedure, influence your willingness or ability to comply with recommendations, and have harmful physical effects on your already weakened physical condition.

We have all experienced the sensation of anxiety at one time or another in our lives. It can feel like a lot of tension in our bodies or a knot in our stomach, or make us apprehensive about a situation. Your heart may begin to race, you may feel sweaty and unable to catch your breath. Your body may shake and leave you feeling weak. Anxiety can stimulate your nervous system, which in turn can increase your chances for experiencing arrhythmias. It can also increase your blood pressure and heart rate. You can see how feeling this way for an extended period of time not only *feels* awful but may physically complicate the recovery process of medical and surgical procedures.

Strategies for Managing Anxiety Related to Medical Procedures

Your current medical condition may require you to undergo several medical or surgical procedures, and although feelings of fear and anxiety are normal they can be managed. Your thoughts are an important part of managing anxiety because they can cause your body to get aroused, which can be a problem when it comes to coping with medical procedures. For instance, if you have the thought that you may bleed to death during the procedure, the sight of any blood may cause you to become anxious and in turn cause your blood pressure to go up and your muscles to tense, which can cause complications during the procedure.

By paying attention to your thoughts and avoiding thinking in black-and-white terms or overgeneralizing situations, you will become better at recognizing what are facts and what are distorted perceptions. Recognition of these false perceptions can help to reduce your pain and anxiety about the procedure. You can use the following strategies to help alleviate any anxiety you might be feeling.

Assess your own style of coping. Coping with or managing anxiety related to medical or surgical procedure is an individual process. Researchers have shown that the most effective coping strategies to reduce anxiety are those that are consistent with a person's usual personality style. For example, some people cope better when given a lot of information and others cope better when they are told very little about the details of the actual procedure. When you are given the amount of information about the procedure that is consistent with your usual style of coping, you are more likely to feel in control, competent to handle the procedure, and as a result, less anxious. What is your usual style of coping? Take the following test to more fully assess your style:

1. Imagine that you are on a plane that is experiencing technical difficulties. Check all of the things you could imagine yourself doing while on the plane.

    _____ Reading a book

    _____ Trying to sleep

    _____ Vigilantly observing the cockpit

    _____ Closely watching the flight attendants facial expressions

    _____ Ordering an alcoholic beverage

    _____ Imagining what your children are doing at that moment

    _____ Closing your eyes and pretending you are on a deserted beach

    _____ Discussing the plane's difficulties with other passengers

    _____ Observing the engine and wings from the window

    _____ Asking the flight attendant every fifteen minutes for an update on the status

2. Imagine that you are giving blood for the first time. Check all of the things you could imagine yourself doing.

_____ Watching the technician to see if he or she puts on clean gloves

_____ Trying to make conversation with the technician about the weather

_____ Inquiring about the procedures for cleaning the area in between donors

_____ Watching the technician insert the needle

_____ Looking in the other direction while the needle is being inserted

_____ Closing your eyes and imagining a quiet scene

_____ Asking the technician to tell you when you would feel a stick of the needle

Did you check more responses that suggest that you like to distract yourself away from the stressful situation? For example, in each of the above situations were you more likely to mentally remove yourself from the situation by imagining something else or distracting yourself with reading or conversation? Or did you check responses that suggest that you need a lot of information and engage in active strategies to cope with the situation, such as asking to be told about possible pain or an update on the events?

Request as much or as little information about the procedure as is consistent with your style of coping. If you are a person who copes better when given information, then ask your physician specific questions before your procedure. Ask questions that will make you feel a part of the procedure and give you a feeling of control. Questions should be specific to sensations that you may experience and the procedure itself. For example:

• What kind of sensations might I experience? A warm feeling over my body? Nausea? Headache? Pressure? Tingling?

• Approximately how long will the procedure take?

• Will I be fully alert?

• Can you talk to me during the procedure and keep me informed?

• Will I feel dull or sharp pain?

• Will I be able to communicate throughout the procedure?

• How many people will be present in the room?

• Will I be able to watch on a monitor?

If, on the other hand, you're a person who copes better by distracting yourself and would rather leave it up to the doctor, then you may need to discuss a strategy of coping with your physician—a strategy that would involve not providing you with *all* of the details related to the procedure. Although legally and ethically medical care providers must give you full and accurate information about procedures, and you must even sign a consent form stating that you fully understand the risks and benefits of the procedure, it doesn't mean that you therefore must hear a blow-by-blow description of the entire procedure and related symptoms that you might experience. Discuss with your doctor your preference to use some distraction techniques to manage your anxiety. This discussion is important because without the support of your doctor, it may be difficult for you to be imagining yourself on a quiet beach while your doctor is talking to you about blood you may see or pain you may experience. Respect for your right to cope in the way that is most comfortable for you is essential for effectively managing anxiety related to a medical procedure.

Use anxiety-producing cues related to the procedure as a trigger for healthy coping strategies. Whether you are a person who needs information to cope or you prefer to distract yourself during stressful events, you can use typical anxiety-producing cues to flip the switch for your individual coping strategy to begin. Many cardiac patients who have undergone a variety of procedures report that certain thoughts, feelings, and cues in the environment can contribute to their anxiety. It is through understanding and being aware of these cues that anxiety can best be managed. These cues may include

- The smell of the room
- The sight of the instruments
- The feeling of a prep sheet on your face or body
- The sound of instruments or voices
- Worries over the staff's competence

These cues or signals may automatically cause you to become anxious without your being aware of it. In a similar fashion, a red light signals you to automatically stop your vehicle. When you see the red signal you automatically, without thought, respond by placing your foot on the brake. In much the same way, without consciously being aware of it, there may be cues or signals related to a past or impending medical procedure that causes you anxiety. The following exercise will help make you more aware of your own personal signals and how you can manage them better:

1. Close your eyes and imagine the procedure. Pay attention to all the things of which you are aware, including sights, sounds, smells, feelings, and thoughts. Identify and list the signals that make you feel uncomfortable. _____

2. In the following chart, briefly list the signals you have identified in the left-hand column. In the right-hand column, change your negative thoughts and cues to positive and realistic thoughts or strategies.

Signal	Positive/Realistic Substitute
Smell of the room	*Trigger to use distraction technique*
Sight of the instrument	*"I know what that will be used for and it looks more frightening than it really is."*

If you are a person who needs information to cope, then use the signal as a cue to engage in dialogue with your physician or simply to talk it through in your head. For example, if the smell of the room triggers anxiety, you might say to yourself, "That smell means that the room is sterile, which means my chances for infection is greatly reduced." On the other hand, if you are a person who needs to distract yourself to effectively cope, then use the smell of the room as a signal for you to go somewhere else in your head. You can use imagery exercises as a way to escape.

3. Rehearse your positive/realistic substitute two times a day for ten minutes.

Use distraction or a relaxation technique. Whether you are a person who likes to be distracted when going through stressful situations or you actively seek out information but like to use relaxation techniques as well, relaxation training may be useful for you.

Relaxation training is a process that helps people learn to improve their ability to concentrate and focus their attention. As you become more relaxed, you may be able to listen better to important things you want to say to yourself. Relaxation training is a self-control technique; *you* are in control, which means that *you* can control your level of relaxation. Like any skill, if you continue to practice you will become better able to relax more fully and in less-than-ideal situations.

Sometimes people wonder if they can get so good at relaxation that they won't be able to respond when they need to. This is impossible. In a relaxed state you can choose to respond when you want to. For example, if your doctor needs you to respond, you can attend to his or her request immediately if you choose to do so.

It is important to realize that in relaxation training you can control how relaxed you get. Try to imagine the scene below, as vividly as possible. The more vividly you try to imagine the scene, the more relaxation you will experience. You may wish to make a tape recording of the following script. Keep the pace slow and steady. You can then listen to the tape in a quiet, relaxed place whenever you wish to practice. Do not listen to the tape while driving.

> Concentrate on your breathing, taking slow, deep breaths. Breathe through your nose, inhale, hold it, exhale slowly. Focus on your belly as it expands like a balloon when you exhale. As you concentrate on slowing down your breathing, also slow down your thinking and let your body relax and sink into a comfortable chair. Notice how relaxed your arms feel against the chair, your legs, your back, and your neck. Notice that your breathing is slow, deep, and regular. You may imagine you are inhaling fresh, clean air, and exhaling all of the tension from your body. Notice how the clean air enters your body and your arms, your legs, your neck, and your back begin to feel relaxed. The tension slowly begins to fade with each exhale.
>
> As you relax, imagine this scene. You are going for a walk in the woods on a beautiful fall day. You enter a forest path and feel the cool shade of many trees. As you walk slowly down the path, notice the trees, underbrush, and fallen branches. Perhaps there is a slightly damp smell of fresh earth and fallen leaves or the deep fragrance of pine. You may hear the crunch of dry leaves under your feet or the rustle of a small friendly animal. Now and then, a bird calls overhead, and you look up to see it gently soaring, sailing skyward. Perhaps you reach over and pick up a stick or a colored leaf, and carry it with you. As you walk on, another pleasant sound begins, at first faintly in the distance, then louder, the clear rushing of water. As you walk on, a clearing appears. As you step into the clearing, you notice that the sun feels warm on your face and a slight breeze gently blows your hair. You notice the sun sparkling on the water of a clear stream. You hear it gurgling as it rushes over the rocks. As you walk toward the stream, you notice a large log lying on the bank, a perfect spot to rest and look at the stream. You may want to sit down for a few moments. Looking in the water, you may see small fish swimming lazily, like colored rocks on the bottom of the beautiful clear stream. You notice how relaxed your body feels.

As you look in the water, feeling more relaxed than you have in a long time, you may feel like taking a few moments to tell yourself some things that are important to you, since this is a time when you are relaxed and better able to listen and concentrate.

(pause for two minutes)

Notice how much more relaxed and comfortable you have become and how much you've enjoyed being in this place. Focus on how relaxed your arms feel, your legs, your neck, your back. In a few minutes you are going to bring yourself back by slowing down your breathing, knowing that you can return to this spot whenever you want.

Now, begin slowing down your breathing while walking down the path. When you are ready, count backwards from five to one. When you reach one, you will open your eyes, feeling relaxed, refreshed, alert, and ready to do what you want to do.

You can use relaxation techniques and imagery exercises to distract yourself during stressful medical procedures, reducing anxiety by redirecting your attention away from the unpleasant experience. Another strategy to distract yourself during the procedure may be bringing in a headset and listening to music or an audiotaped version of a favorite book.

PART 2

Adjustment
Immediately after
a Heart Attack

Heart attacks occur so often because people wrongly believe someone else will get them.

—Eduardo Chapunoff, M.D.

4

Heart Attack: What If
It Happens to You?

What Happens after a
Heart Attack?

If you've had a heart attack and arrived at the emergency room, you may expect the following general course of events: The actual diagnosis of myocardial infarction will be made by a physician who has reviewed results of several tests. The physician will review your complete medical history and perform a physical examination. An EKG will be given to examine any abnormalities caused by damage to your heart. A blood test measuring levels of enzymes in your blood that rise when heart muscle is damaged is also usually done.

If a diagnosis of a heart attack is confirmed, therapy with thrombolytic, or clot-dissolving, drugs may be started if your symptoms began no more than a few hours earlier and if your doctor determines this type of drug could help restore blood flow to your heart. The medication may be started in the emergency room or in the intensive care unit, depending upon the practices of your hospital. You will likely be placed in an intensive care unit or coronary care unit of the hospital. Here, you will be continuously monitored by EKG as well as by regular checks of important vital signs, like blood pressure and heart rate.

Additional tests will probably be performed during your hospitalization to determine the extent of blockage in your coronary arteries. Tests may include EKGs at rest and during exercise, with or without some type of heart scan, and possibly coronary angiography or echocardiography. The purpose of the tests is to identify the amount of damage to your heart muscle caused by the attack and whether or not treatments such as CABG or balloon angioplasty may be necessary to treat narrowed or blocked arteries.

In making decisions about which treatments are recommended for you, your doctor will take into account your general health, age, test results, and various other issues. Conventional treatments used for heart attacks include painkillers for any ongoing pain associated with the attack; aspirin to make your blood less sticky; and possibly medications such as anticoagulants, which reduce risks of blood clots forming.

Two out of three people who have heart attacks will survive and recover. If the damaged area of the heart is small and does not lead to dangerous changes in your heart's rate or rhythm, the attack should not be fatal and your chances of making a good recovery are improved. Most deaths from heart attacks occur within minutes or up to two hours from the time symptoms began. So if you've made it this far, you can relax—your chances of surviving this heart attack are good.

Complications that can occur after a heart attack include the following:

- About 10 percent of patients admitted to hospitals with heart attacks go into shock, which can be fatal. Because the heart is not pumping blood efficiently, the flow of blood throughout the body suddenly drops, and vital body organs cannot function well. If not treated promptly, the body's vital organs may die from lack of oxygen.

- The heart can react to a blockage in a coronary artery by generating *ventricular fibrillation* (an irregular rhythm). When this happens, the heart muscle flutters so rapidly that it can't produce good contractions. And without these, the heart fails to pump any blood at all (cardiac arrest). Unless this irregular heart rhythm is corrected quickly, the heart can stop beating completely within seconds to minutes.

- Another risk after heart attack, though rare—occurring in only about 5 percent of cases—is an *embolism*. This happens when a blood clot that forms inside the heart breaks loose into the circulatory system, where it can travel and cause damage in other parts of the body.

- Blood clots may form in the veins, most often in the legs.

- Heart failure may occur if damage from the heart attack leads to weakening or stretching of the heart chambers.

If you experience any of these complications, then your recovery may be somewhat slower and more difficult.

Studies suggest that if you're alive one month or more after even a severe attack, you have a 70 to 80 percent chance of surviving for at least five years. However, most episodes of cardiac arrest occur within eighteen months after being discharged from the hospital for a heart attack. Because of this, family members of heart attack survivors should consider getting training in CPR.

Although in the past, heart attack patients were kept as still as possible for extended time periods, current practices encourage as much activity as permitted given the patients' physical condition. Doctors now believe that moving around as soon as possible lowers the risk of abnormal blood clotting. When first admitted to the hospital, you can expect at least a short period of bed rest (about twelve hours). If you don't have complications, you will probably be allowed light activities such as going to the bathroom, assisted bathing, and slow walking after this rest period. You will also be given a drug called heparin, which thins out your blood and further reduces your chances for developing blood clots.

Based upon your test results, your doctor may prescribe long-term drug therapy to reduce strain on your heart, improve your heart's efficiency, or prevent irregular heart rhythms from occurring. Prior to your discharge from the hospital, a stress EKG may be performed to provide information about how much exercise is safe for you. In addition, your doctor will also recommend that you enroll in a cardiac rehabilitation program, which assists you with exercise as well as controlling other risk factors like weight, smoking, and stress.

Sometimes after a heart attack, survivors experience changes in mental status or thinking processes. Examples of this include confusion, disorientation, problems with memory, or even hallucinations. Such changes, often reflecting a condition called *delirium*, can be related to side effects of heart medications, complications of the heart attack, or a variety of physical disorders. The medical staff will likely identify these changes quickly. But if you are a family member of a heart patient and notice any such changes, tell the staff immediately. These problems can be treated successfully, but sometimes reflect a serious complication that requires prompt treatment. Additionally, it's important to recognize any difficulties with thought processes, because if the problems persist, they can interfere with understanding, remembering, and following medical recommendations.

Coping with Anxiety in the Hospital

A heart attack is a profound emotional, as well as physical, event. Your fears about potential death and real or imagined losses can change your outlook on life forever. These changes in outlook and lifestyle may actually enrich and improve the quality of your life. However, a struggle with anxiety, depression, or loss of self-confidence can lead to physical limitations and poorer health, family conflicts, job insecurities, and sexual problems.

The most obvious and immediate response to a heart attack is anxiety. Upon learning that you have had a heart attack, it's normal to have fears of disability or death. Any ongoing pain from the heart attack will also tend to increase your anxiety levels. In addition, simply being in an intensive care unit can be a nerve-wracking experience. The highly technical setting, sounds of monitoring equipment, frequent checks by medical staff, and possible calls of "Code Blue" for neighboring patients can contribute to heightened states of anxiety and worry. Unfortunately, the body's response to anxiety generally involves the cardiovascular system with responses such as increased heart rate and blood pressure and increased stickiness of blood. So not only is anxiety a miserable emotional state, but it's also a physically dangerous side effect for someone who already has a vulnerable heart. Keep in mind, though, that some degree of fear is good. It can prompt you to make changes in your life that can be emotionally and physically beneficial. Occasional anxiety is not harmful. But prolonged, chronic anxiety is miserable and destructive to your heart. If you have high levels of stress while in the hospital, you may be three times more likely to die within the next five years than those with low levels of stress (Frasure-Smith 1991).

To control any ongoing pain, medications such as morphine may be given. Often, these painkillers alleviate anxiety as well. Be open and specific in informing the medical staff when pain occurs. Rating your pain using a number scale from 1 to 10 can be helpful to you and the staff in following your progress. Don't wait for pain to become severe before asking for medications. Short-term use of narcotics for pain control is not addicting. Good control of pain is necessary for good recovery.

Anxiety in cardiac patients may be expressed in a variety of ways. You may appear overtly distressed, overly sensitive or vigilant to what's happening around you, or you may have a sense of dread or foreboding. You may feel restless, distractible, tense, irritable, or easily startled. You may have difficulties sleeping. Physical signals of anxiety may include increased heart rate, sweating, shortness of breath, and high blood pressure. On the other hand, you may be quietly watchful and seemingly unconcerned about your condition. This may reflect a kind of avoidance or denial. Though denial on a long-term basis may interfere with making necessary changes in lifestyle, in an immediate sense, it can offer some benefits.

The best advice for you during your hospital stay may be to do what comes naturally. When coping with stressful situations, some people tend to use avoidance strategies. This means that you do not want to be overwhelmed with detailed information and would rather distract yourself, focusing on more pleasant thoughts in the heat of stressful moments. If this sounds like you, trying to focus too much on the details of what's happening around you can increase your anxiety. To stay as calm as possible, your best approach may be to limit information only to what is essential. Keep in mind, though, that after your discharge and during recovery, it's important to process carefully all that has happened to you and what has been recommended in terms of lifestyle changes. Otherwise, denial can lead to avoidance of changes that can improve the quality of your life as well as your cardiac health.

Others tend to cope with stress by actively seeking information. This means that you feel more comfortable and in control when you have detailed facts about what has happened and what will happen to you. If this is your style, ask a lot of questions and get specific information to put your mind at rest. However, to avoid becoming overly preoccupied with thoughts or worries that increase anxiety, limit the time you spend on this. For example, when a question occurs to you, write it down and then try to stop thinking about it until you can speak with your doctor. Be sure to spend some time relaxing as much as possible. Activities like reading or watching television can distract you from concerns about your health.

The medical staff will monitor your emotional state as well as physical status during your stay in the hospital. However, sometimes the focus is more on your physical recovery—to the neglect of your emotional adjustment. This is especially true if your response to anxiety is subtle and does not lead to easily recognizable, overt signs in your behavior. If this is the case, you should be open and direct in describing your anxiety to the medical staff. Also, if you've had struggles with anxiety in the past, let your doctor know about this as well. This is important not only for your emotional well-being, but because emotional distress may interfere with cardiac healing and can even contribute to complications. In response to anxiety, the body releases chemicals or stress hormones, such as adrenaline and cortisol. These stress hormones can affect blood clotting, make your blood stickier, cause a greater strain on the pumping of your heart, or lead to irregular heart rhythms.

Once your physician has become aware of your anxiety levels, he or she will probably rule out any physical cause for the anxiety. Some heart medications can have anxiety symptoms as a side effect. In addition, some physical conditions, such as thyroid imbalance, can contribute to anxiety symptoms. If you were a smoker prior to your hospitalization, symptoms of nicotine withdrawal can include anxiety, as well as insomnia, depression, difficulty concentrating, irritability, restlessness, and slowed heart rate. Be sure to inform your doctor about smoking habits. Additionally, if you were a regular or heavy drinker of alcohol (more than two drinks per day), tell your physician about this as well. Your body may experience withdrawal symptoms, possibly including anxiety symptoms, from the lack of alcohol.

After considering the causes for your anxiety, your doctor may prescribe an anti-anxiety medication. Additionally, you can improve your adjustment by learning a better response to stress. Here are some techniques you can use in the hospital to reduce anxious feelings and thereby assist in your physical recovery:

- Try to spend some time **relaxing.** Though this can be difficult in a setting as hectic as an intensive care unit, distracting yourself by reading, watching television, or listening to music may be helpful. If you already have a favorite relaxation exercise, such as deep breathing, use it. Slow, quiet music may have a calming, relaxing effect. Researchers have found that music influences heart rate, breathing rate, blood pressure, and hormone levels. Studies of the coronary intensive care unit have indicated that music may decrease rapid, irregular heart rates, lower blood pressure, increase pain tolerance, and reduce anxiety levels (Guzzetta 1989; White 1992).

- Engage in **positive thinking.** Don't allow your thoughts to increase your anxiety and concerns about your health. Replace negative thoughts with positive, reassuring statements.

Negative Thoughts	Positive Reassurance
I feel so helpless; there's nothing I can do.	*I can and will get through this.*
I can't stand this pain.	*The discomfort will pass.*
I'll never get better. What if I die?	*I'm alive now and recovering. I will recover and be strong again.*

  Repeating statements such as "My breathing is calm and regular" and "My heart rate is calm and regular" can assist in lowering anxiety and relaxing the body.

- Rely on **support** of family and friends. Having a good network of family and friends is associated with a better recovery after a heart attack.

- **Consult** with a mental health professional (psychologist, psychiatrist, or social worker). This option is available to you at most hospitals. Psychological support provided to heart attack survivors during hospitalization can help diminish anxiety and depression, decrease length of hospital stays, and decrease risk of complications. If your attempts to control anxiety on your own do not feel sufficient, feel free to ask your doctor for a psychological consultation.

Research has indicated that your beliefs about your heart attack and its consequences have a major effect on how well you will adjust and recover. For example, heart attack survivors with a more optimistic outlook about their illness tend to return to work faster than those who believe their illness will cause permanent disability (Scheier et al. 1989). If you are a positive thinker, you may be more likely to make heart-healthy changes in your lifestyle and follow through with medical advice than others with more pessimistic outlooks.

Coping with Depression in the Hospital

After a heart attack, fears of disability and concerns about being normal or strong again can lead to depression. Signs of depression include

- Feelings of sadness or irritability
- Lack of energy and motivation
- Reduced enjoyment of activities
- Problems concentrating
- Decreased sexual drive
- Feelings of hopelessness or helplessness that may lead to thoughts of suicide

In general, persons with heart disease appear more likely to be depressed. Estimated rates of depression in various groups of heart patients are about 30 percent: this is four to five times greater than rates of depression in the general population. If you had problems with depression prior to hospitalization, this may have even contributed to your heart attack. More and more studies are showing a recurring link between depression and the development of heart disease. If you already have coronary heart disease, your chances of future heart problems, like a recurrent heart attack, are greater if you are depressed. People who are depressed also appear less able to effectively control behaviors that lead to risk factors for heart disease, such as overeating and smoking.

If you've had past struggles with feeling depressed, even if you've never been treated for depression, tell your physician about this. Depression may be caused by a number of physical conditions (such as thyroid imbalance), as well as medication side effects. Grief is a normal part of adjusting to any serious medical illness such as a heart attack. It's when feelings of depression are chronic and severe that they seem to be most damaging to your physical and emotional well-being.

While in the hospital, you can exert some control over depression by using the techniques discussed for relieving anxiety. Getting detailed information in terms of what to expect during your recovery is crucial and can be a big help in challenging fears you may have. Ask your doctor detailed questions about how to approach your life at home after discharge from the hospital. General issues to question include work, exercise, and sexual activity. Use the following sample questions as a guide:

- When can I go back to work?
- Should I change my work schedule or reduce my regular work hours?
- How will my job be affected by my heart condition?
- Should I avoid any particular work-related activities?
- When should I begin exercising?
- What kind of exercises can I do, and for how long can I exercise at a time?
- What are the signs that should tell me to stop exercising?
- How will my heart condition, and my heart medications, affect my sex life? When can I resume sexual activities with my partner?
- Are there any sexual activities or positions I should avoid?
- When should I take my medications (in relation to timing for sexual activities)?
- What if I have chest pains during sex?
- When can I drive or travel by air?

If you become depressed after a heart attack, or if you struggled with depression before your heart attack, it's crucial to get help for this. Not only does depression affect the quality of your life, but it can have a negative impact on your recovery. Many studies have shown poorer recovery rates and greater likelihood of future heart problems in people with untreated depression. In a study of heart attack survivors, depression was more closely related to future heart problems than the degree of artery blockage, high cholesterol, or cigarette smoking (Frasure-Smith et al. 1995). If you have survived a heart attack, depression may triple your risk of dying within three months. The good news is that treatment for depression is associated with improved chances of survival and reduced risks of future heart problems.

What to Expect during Your Recovery

If you're reading this after surviving a heart attack, then your chances of recovery are good. Predictions about your recovery depend on factors like your age, medical history, type of heart attack, and complications you may have had. In general, if you are alive one month after even a severe attack, you have a 70 to 80 percent chance of surviving for at least five years. However, you will probably need to make some significant changes in your lifestyle in order to speed your recovery and slow down—or maybe even reverse—the heart disease you have. Behaviors you may have to change include exercise, diet, smoking, following through with taking medications, and managing stress levels.

Making lifestyle changes, which will be addressed in part 3, may be easier for you to achieve if you participate in a structured cardiac rehabilitation program. These programs combine exercise training with education about ways you can change behaviors that increase your risks for heart disease. Cardiac rehabilitation programs can offer the following benefits:

- Improve your capacity for physical activity
- Reduce chances of dying from heart disease
- Reverse atherosclerosis (buildup of plaque in your arteries, leading to narrower passages for blood flow)
- Reduce your risk of having future heart attacks
- Improve the quality of your life
- Make you more likely to comply with your doctor's recommendations
- Lessen emotional distress
- Lessen unhealthy denial

In spite of these findings, only about 15 percent of qualified patients actually participate in cardiac rehabilitation programs. This may be due to a number of factors, such as lack of referral by physicians, poor motivation of patients, and financial or technical difficulties (like transportation problems). If your doctor recommended a rehabilitation program for you, do yourself a favor: try it. If you didn't get a referral from your doctor, then ask why not. There are some home exercise training programs that may be beneficial for you as an alternative to structured cardiac rehabilitation. But with the home programs, you miss out on the ability to interact with others and get the information provided by the cardiac rehabilitation group program.

Recent studies have suggested that when treatments geared toward helping with emotional and/or social difficulties are included in the cardiac rehabilitation programs, results are even better (Linden et al. 1996). These therapies are often referred to as *psychosocial treatments*, and include individual or group counseling, relaxation training, music therapy, or changing negative thought and behavior patterns. Being involved in such comprehensive programs has been associated with decreased risks of dying, reduced chance of a recurrent heart attack, reduced emotional distress, improved quality of life, and even improvements in traditional medical risk factors like blood pressure, heart rate, and cholesterol levels. Researchers suggest that psychosocial treatments should be routinely included in cardiac rehabilitation programs. Especially if you have struggled with anxiety or depression, ask your doctor about programs that include these components. You can also seek your own psychological treatment through individual or group counseling. Ask your doctor or friends for referrals.

Your doctor will make specific recommendations that apply to your case with regard to returning to work. Unless changes are suggested by your doctor, there is no evidence that taking a less responsible job or working part-time will help your health. The American Heart Association (Ryan et al. 1996) reports that return-to-work rates for heart attack patients range from 63 to 94 percent. Keep in mind that these rates are influenced by factors other than health status, such as job satisfaction, financial stability, and company policies. Return to prior levels of activity is probably a better gauge of recovery.

If you had an uncomplicated heart attack and do not have symptoms such as angina afterward, you can very likely return to your prior activities within two weeks. Talk with your doctor about the safety of specific activities you have in mind. Again, being involved in a cardiac rehabilitation program is a good way to gain confidence in your abilities at a variety of levels of physical exercise. You can usually begin with daily walking immediately after discharge from the hospital. If your condition is stable and without complications, you can usually gradually resume sexual activities within a few weeks after your discharge. When you can return to driving after a serious illness is regulated by guidelines established by your state's Department of Motor Vehicles. You can usually resume driving within one to two weeks of your discharge. Certain restrictions, such as avoiding stressful situations like rush hour, bad weather, night driving, heavy traffic, and high speeds, may initially apply. The American Heart Association suggests that within the first two weeks after discharge from the hospital, only patients who are stable, do not have a fear of flying, and who travel with a companion should travel by air.

When approaching your life after your heart attack, you may find that you have difficulty making needed changes in your lifestyle. Your personality makeup may lead you to deny the significance of the attack and stay stuck in old, habitual, self-destructive patterns of behavior. But many people benefit from having had such a serious, life-threatening event. A New Zealand study surveyed patients recovering from either heart attacks or breast cancer treatment (Petrie et al. 1996). The researchers found that many persons saw their illness as an opportunity to reevaluate what was really important in their lives. Over half of those surveyed reported healthy lifestyle changes. Almost one-third said they have a greater appreciation of life and health. And about one-fourth described improved close relationships. You, too, can use your experience as an opportunity to make changes in your life that perhaps you have never thought possible before.

Dr. Robert Eliot (1984), who himself had a heart attack, suggests that the most important question you can answer for yourself in your recovery is, "Why did I have a heart attack now?" Dr. Eliot suggests that knowing the reasons for your attack gives you most of the knowledge you need to prevent another heart attack. What was your life like in the months prior to your attack? How did you cope with the stresses in your life? Many heart attack survivors describe having lived—often for many years—under high levels of stress. They also report feeling overwhelmed, discouraged, and defeated in their attempts to overcome their stresses. As mentioned previously, a sudden emotional upset or episode is often an immediate trigger for a heart attack. After you've identified what likely contributed to your heart attack, you have more power to change heart-destructive behaviors. Reflect on your priorities, and do some reorganizing of them if necessary.

If you've never had a heart attack or other life-threatening illness, don't wait for such a crisis to spur you to make changes. Acting now can prevent future heart difficulties and improve the quality and enjoyment of life.

5

When Your Loved One Has Had a Heart Attack: For Partners and Family Members

This chapter will address the adjustment issues that face the partners and family members of the heart attack patient. The endless barrage of stressors, including feelings of loss of control, dependence on the doctors and medical staff at the hospital, disruption of the day-to-day lifestyle, worry about the future, and fears of suffering and death and so on, are also many of the same stressors experienced by the family, especially the partner of the heart attack victim. While the patient understandably receives the most attention, reassurance, support, and treatment as needed to help with the fear and anxiety, family members are often left to struggle with their fears and stress without any support. The changes that will be facing the patient will also result in changes that the family must make. For instance, during the period immediately following a heart attack, the spouse or partner may have to assume the responsibilities of both people in the household, such as earning an income, doing all of the household duties, paying the bills, and parenting any children if there are children living at home. This is an overwhelming task, especially when the partner is simultaneously trying to cope with all of his or her own set of fears. Therefore, adjusting to a heart attack is a family affair. The success of the heart attack patient's adjustment and cardiac rehabilitation may be dependent, in part, on the family's participation.

The Family Member's Experience in the Coronary Care Unit

Whether you were present to witness your loved one's heart attack or whether you received a call, the immediate reaction is one of shock and numbness. You may recall racing to the hospital emergency room and, in dazed confusion, being directed to the coronary care waiting room, where you sat and waited for some news of what happened. Simply waiting may have felt extremely stressful because of the fear of the unknown. The last time you spoke with your loved one might be replayed vividly in your mind. If you saw the person unconscious, the fear of him or her dying may have been terrifying. When the physician came out to speak with you, you may not even recall the exact words spoken except, "Your husband (or your wife, father, and so on) has had a heart attack." Issues such as treatment, chances of a good recovery, and a myriad of other questions become a blur at this time.

The coronary care unit (CCU) is a specialized unit focused on providing acute care to the patient who has suffered a heart attack. The functioning of the heart is observed carefully through heart monitors and the unit is staffed with trained doctors and nurses twenty-four hours a day. Visiting hours are strictly controlled and limited to one-hour time periods in most CCUs so as not to unduly disturb the patient. Therefore, family members often sit in the CCU waiting room for an opportunity to see their loved one and to have some contact with the medical staff. This can leave them feeling helpless and anxious. The first time you saw your sick spouse or relative after the heart attack or surgery, with tubes and monitors hooked up to various parts of their body, may have aroused intense feelings of helplessness, panic, and sadness. If you had this experience, it is normal and even expected that you found yourself having intense feelings of fear, confusion and frustration, and you may have behaved in ways that were out of character for you. For instance, you may have been very irritable and demanding of the medical staff, or you may have sat in the waiting room and simply cried. Any reaction that you may have experienced can be thought of as a normal reaction to a crisis.

Think back to the time period when you first heard that your spouse, parent, or other family member had a heart attack and answer the following questions.

If you were with the person when the heart attack happened, what did you do? (Did you have to call 911? Did you administer CPR? Did you feel paralyzed and not know what to do?)

Was your loved one conscious or unconscious? Did you talk with him or her?

Did you ride in the ambulance or did you have to follow in another car? What do you remember feeling?

When you arrived at the hospital, what was your experience like? What do you recall feeling?

If you were not present when the person had his or her heart attack, where were you?

What do you recall feeling about not being present?

Sharing your feelings with your family and friends will help you cope with this overwhelming experience. Keeping it all inside by pretending that it will go away or minimizing your feelings will not be helpful to you or anyone else. Talking about traumatic events soon after they have occurred can help prevent a more serious reaction at a later date. Grief is a normal reaction to a traumatic event that has changed your life. For most people, the heart attack came with little or no warning and thus there was no time to prepare for the consequences afterwards. You may find yourself crying, not sleeping well, eating too little or too much, having trouble concentrating, or feeling very sad. Usually, a grief reaction to the illness is time-limited, especially as you start to see your loved one recover and participate in rehabilitation. Remember that your spouse or family member will need a lot of support and encouragement from you at this time. So it's important to take care of yourself by getting support from others and also by communicating with your spouse or family member. Better communication will only improve your relationship and draw you closer.

It's often helpful to have a list of questions prepared for the doctors when they speak with you about the patient's status. It's not unusual to feel so distraught or numb that it becomes difficult to focus on what the doctor is saying or asking. If your partner or family member is too ill, you may be asked to make important medical decisions regarding treatment. Although the choices for treating your loved one may be limited (that is, it may be necessary to do a CABG to prevent an another heart attack immediately), you may still have to give consent. The presence of another family member or friend can be helpful to you. Write down what the doctor says so that you can refer to the information later. The following questions can serve as a guide:

- Will you explain what has happened? Perhaps you could draw a diagram. What is the amount and type of damage to the heart?

- What risks or potential immediate concerns do you have? For instance, is he or she in danger of having another heart attack immediately?

- What type of treatments are being given? What are the advantages and disadvantages of each type of treatment and how will you go about treating my family member? What are the chances of the artery closing up again soon after a procedure such as balloon angioplasty versus a coronary artery bypass graft surgery?

- Where can I get reference books on heart disease so that I may begin to educate myself?

Other members of the medical team, such as nurses, social workers, and psychologists, can also be helpful to you. They are available to give you more information themselves, or they can direct you to the appropriate resources. For example, if you have financial concerns, such as insurance coverage, one of the medical staff may be able to help find the information that you need. Finally, an excellent source of support in the CCU waiting room are spouses and family members of the other patients. They too are experiencing many of the same issues you are facing. While every case is unique, and the information that applies to their loved one may not be pertinent to yours, they are nonetheless a valuable resource. Often spouses and family members feel that they have to put up a strong front for the benefit of their hospitalized loved one, but they can more easily share their fears and concerns with other spouses and families experiencing the same thing.

The Coping Patterns of Families

Families will cope with the cardiac illness of a loved one in a variety of ways, some healthy and some unhealthy. The patterns of coping are determined, in part, by the way in which the family members related prior to the heart attack. All families have their own style of interacting with each other. Family therapists liken this to a team or a system where each person in the family has a role that seems to just naturally occur without any conscious thought. For example, one member of the family may be the peacemaker who soothes conflict and tension between other family members. Another person may be the caretaker, always attending to everyone's needs. Yet a third person may be the baby of the family and used to being treated as such.

Another characteristic of families is the "rules" of the family. These rules may be unspoken or spoken and often dictate how each member relates to one another. These rules may include how emotions are expressed, how conflict and arguments are handled, and what are the values and beliefs of the family. In a couple, each person will bring the rules of his or her own family of origin to a relationship. The way in which the couple relate to each other also sets the tone for their children. Virginia Satir (1972), a well-known family therapist, believed that the marital relationship is the central core around which the other family relationships are formed. If the couple relates to each other in a healthy manner, then the other family relationships will also be healthy.

What were some the characteristics of your family of origin, that is, the family in which you grew up? For instance, were emotions discussed openly or was everyone expected to be strong? Did your parents fight openly or only behind closed doors? Did conflicts between themselves or between you and them get resolved or were they left to fester inside?

_____

_____

What was your role in your family of origin? For example, were you the peacemaker, troublemaker, caretaker, baby?

_____

Similarly, what are some of the ways in which your own family (partner and children, if you have any) related before the heart attack? For instance, were you in charge? How did you communicate? Did you keep an emotional distance?

_____

_____

Unhealthy Coping Styles

The stress accompanying a heart attack can disturb the way family members relate to one another. The patterns that develop after the heart attack can often be unhealthy, and in turn, may be detrimental to the health of everyone in the family. It's usually easier to detect when the heart patient is in distress than to recognize that a family member is not doing well. The patient naturally receives a lot of attention from the family and the health care team, and poor coping can be easily seen by indicators such as depression, low motivation to participate in rehabilitation, irritability, and anxiety. Family members also have reactions to the illness, but their problems with adjustment are not always easy to see. For example, it can sometimes appear on the surface that you are adjusting well to your partner's illness because neither you nor your family are not showing any obvious signs of distress. But a family can gradually become distressed over time in response to the multiple changes caused by a heart attack.

Following are examples of signs of distress to look for in yourself if your partner or someone else in your family has had a heart attack. You may find that you have experienced a few of these already during your own adjustment process. Staying stuck in a particular mode can lead to unhealthy relationships in your family and tension within yourself.

Physical symptoms. If you already have health problems of your own, these may worsen at the time that your partner or family member has a heart attack. Periods of stress can exacerbate your own problems, and the added strain may mean that you are not taking as good care of yourself. It's also not unusual to experience other physical symptoms such as chest palpitations, sleep and appetite problems, headaches, and stomach upset as a result of stress. If these symptoms do not improve after a few days, please see your doctor. If you are experiencing chest pain or discomfort or difficulty breathing, it's important to have yourself checked out immediately, even if you think it's nothing significant. You may be tempted to ignore your own symptoms because someone else is acutely ill and needs you, but it's important to take care of yourself as well in times of crisis.

Depression. When the grief reaction appears to be lasting too long, depression can be the cause. Persistent problems with your mood (feeling low), appetite, sleep, and concentration may be a sign that you are depressed. If the heart attack has significantly changed the roles so that you must now take care of everything while your partner or family member is recovering, you can be easily overwhelmed. This can lead to depression, especially if your own needs are not being met for a significant period of time. It will be important to seek help if you find that you are depressed. Heart disease is a lifelong illness and as such will require commitment to lifestyle changes. Life may never be the same as it was prior to the heart attack. If these changes lead to feelings of depression for you, seek professional help by speaking to a mental health professional who is familiar with issues related to adjustment to illness. For further reading on depression and the distinction between depression and normal adjustment reaction, refer to chapter 12.

Denial of the illness. For some family members the threat of illness and possible loss of their loved one becomes too frightening, so they cope by pretending that their spouse or parent is not that sick. They may minimize any symptoms by saying, "It's just indigestion" or "It's nothing serious" or "High cholesterol runs in the family and nothing has happened yet." They may often join the person with the heart problem in denying or minimizing potentially serious problems instead of urging the patient to seek help or change important risk factors. Another way of denying the illness is to not participate in cardiac rehabilitation, where they can learn about heart disease. Denial of the seriousness of cardiac illness can be life-threatening. It can lead to delay in seeking treatment when experiencing symptoms of a heart attack as well as make it difficult for the patient to make the necessary lifestyle changes. If you have been minimizing the warnings given by the doctor, seek assistance to help determine the reasons. Addressing the issues head-on will be healthier for you and your loved one in the long run.

Guilt. As part of the myriad of emotions you will feel during this adjustment period, feelings of guilt can be present and sometimes debilitating. Family members may feel guilty because they were arguing with their loved one when the heart attack occurred or because they fear that they unknowingly ignored warning signs of an impending heart attack. For example, your spouse may have looked unusually pale and tired for a couple of days prior to the heart attack, but you may have pushed to get some household chore finished anyway. It is not unusual to hear family members say, "I didn't tell him that I loved him" or "I wish that I didn't argue with her last week" or "I should have seen this coming." If you've felt intense anger towards your partner due to problems in the relationship, you may feel guilty now that he or she is ill. For some people who are in an abusive relationship, the intense anger that develops as a result of the abuse can lead to some prior fantasies of revenge or of their spouse or family member dying. When the abuser gets a heart attack, the abused may feel guilt about having "wished it to happen." Whatever the circumstances at the time the heart attack happened, it's unlikely that your actions actually *caused* the heart attack. While it is true that stress contributes to heart disease, there are also several other factors that contribute and likely caused the heart attack to occur. Holding on to feelings of guilt and ceasing to communicate effectively with your partner for fear of causing another heart attack will not be healthy. Focus instead on communicating your fears to your spouse or family member directly. You might even try to address the problems in your relationship either by sitting down with your spouse or family member or by seeking counseling.

Anger. Persistent anger about the changes that the heart attack has brought to your life can also be damaging. It's true that heart disease is a lifelong illness and the additional roles you may have to take over can lead to feelings of resentment. Increased irritability, moodiness, temper outbursts, and snapping at others are signs of anger at having to cope with the new demands. This anger can also be directed towards the medical staff for not "doing enough" and may lead to strained relationships with the very people that are needed to provide support and consistent medical care. If you find that you're angry and resentful on many occasions, take a break and examine some of the reasons why. There may be other options available to you that will ease some of the demands. By using effective communication and some problem-solving skills, you can reduce the level of anger that you feel. Some of these strategies are presented in chapter 15. Remaining angry all of the time is a risk factor for developing heart disease of your own.

Overworking and overprotectiveness. Sometimes family members and partners feel that they have to do everything to take care of their sick loved one. They attempt to alleviate all of the stress the person is experiencing by taking over all of the responsibilities of the household, the finances, child rearing, and so on so that they can protect their loved one from experiencing *any* stress and therefore prevent another heart attack. This, of course, can occur for only a certain period of time before the overworked family member or partner becomes fatigued, depressed, burned out, and even resentful. The overprotected person can also feel depressed because he or she seems to have lost all control of his or her everyday life. You may find that indeed you must take over all of the responsibilities while your loved one is recovering. But continuing to shield him or her from all stress can become stressful in itself, both for your spouse and for you, and it will not necessarily prevent another heart attack from happening, because there are multiple risk factors. As the person continues to recover, he or she will be able to gradually get back into life's activities. Cardiac rehabilitation will assist you and your spouse or family member in returning to normal functioning. Learning to cope effectively with life's stressors is part of the rehabilitation process and is necessary to help reduce the risk of another heart attack.

Walking on eggshells. This is a variation of overprotecting the sick loved one. Many heart attack patients have personality styles that include getting angry, blowing up, and general impatience over everyday matters. For fear that they will have another heart attack, spouses and family members often learn to hold their own feelings in so as not to provoke the sick person. If you find yourself adjusting your thoughts, feelings, and actions and walking on eggshells, you can soon find yourself resentful and depressed. Communicating your needs in a calm but assertive manner and helping your partner or family member hear you without getting angry or upset can help reduce your tension and help the family communicate with more honesty and closeness. These factors, in turn, can promote recovery for the heart patient.

Withdrawal from each other. This can be described as a passive withdrawal from life as a response to stress and fear. Some families have already established a pattern in which each member sort of takes care of him- or herself. In times of crises like an illness, remaining distant from each other can create more stress and leave each person to cope with the new demands on their own. As you will read about in chapter 13, social isolation has been linked with increased chances of having another heart attack in people with previously diagnosed heart disease. Poor emotional connections in the family can also lead to feelings of depression and anger because one's needs are not being met during this period of stress. Once again, learning to communicate your feelings effectively to your sick partner or family member, even if you are not used to this, is healthier for you, your sick loved one, and the rest of your family.

Healthy Coping Styles

If you've identified with any of the unhealthy coping styles, the most effective solution is to have open communication about your needs, feelings, and concerns. Successful adjustment to the heart attack requires participation from all involved. While no marriage, relationship, or family is perfect, some are successful with their adjustment during periods of crisis and come out of them with increased closeness. Some of these guidelines may help you and your partner or family member cope with the adjustment to heart disease:

- During the acute phase of the illness, recognize that your sick loved one may feel too overwhelmed, tired, and ill to participate in many discussions with anyone. Therefore, if he or she appears withdrawn and unresponsive to you, try not take it personally— allow your partner to get his or her bearings slowly. Lean on others for support and if you find yourself becoming too angry and frustrated with everyone, including the medical staff, ask to speak to a mental health professional. They cannot take away the real pain of what has happened, but they can assist you with coping during this acute crisis.

- As your loved one begins to recover, share some of your feelings and concerns about him or her and your life together. You might have heard the myth that heart patients should be protected from dealing with strong emotions. But shielding the person from expressing him- or herself and hearing you honestly will only isolate the both of you and, in turn, be unhealthy and more stressful for the heart.

- Join together to gather as much information as possible about the heart attack, aspects of rehabilitation, and the lifestyle changes that will need to be made. Continue to monitor each other and be supportive of each others' fears and frustrations. This time is full of adjustment and loss. Now would also be the time to consider joining your loved one in some of the lifestyle changes, such as diet or exercise. It will be easier if the both of you are doing things together.

- Limit statements of concerns to those that begin with "I feel" and stay away from blaming and accusations. Even if you're angry at the person for ignoring your warnings and continuing with a stressful, unhealthy lifestyle, throwing blame will only alienate you both.

- Try to approach the new changes in your roles with flexibility. You may feel initially resentful and overburdened, but with time, your partner or family member will be able to assume more responsibility. Remaining rigid in what you used to do versus what you *have* to do now will only increase tension.

- Gather as much social support around you as possible. Get or maintain some outside interests that will keep you both stimulated and distracted from the stress of coping with the illness.

- Continue open dialogue with your loved one with each new phase of adjustment. View this period as an opportunity to become closer instead of becoming lonely and isolated.

Special Needs of Children

If your spouse has had a heart attack and there are children still living at home, the children may show their distress in a variety of ways. Because the initial focus of attention is justifiably on the heart patient, often children can be left feeling confused, frightened, and lost. Their ultimate fear is, naturally, losing a parent. If you've been thinking that openly talking to your child about heart disease will only further distress him or her, please reconsider. Children almost always are aware of what is going on but often are not yet skilled in expressing their feelings. Their fears must be addressed from the onset in order to prevent problems in their own development. You can talk to your child either as a couple or separately, but the sick parent need not be isolated from communicating with his or her children. The following are some signs that your child or teenager is in distress:

- Trouble sleeping, or frequent awakening at night
- Nightmares

- Appetite changes

- Acting sullen or withdrawn

- Frequent temper outbursts

- Complaints of physical symptoms, like headaches, stomachaches

- Drop in school performance

- Behavioral problems, like fighting and lying

- Fear of being separated from parent, particularly the sick one

- Drug or alcohol use

- Persistent fears and worries

The following guidelines can help you talk to your children about coping with a parent's illness:

- Ask your children how they are feeling about what has happened. Be sure to address and hear from all of your children. Sometimes you may have one child who appears to be doing better than the others but is actually keeping distress inside. Even if your child says nothing, talk anyway. Children usually absorb more than they let on.

- Answer any questions they may have regarding the heart disease. Try to explain in terms they can understand (age appropriate), or with pictures, what a heart attack is. Reassure them that the parent is receiving good medical care and that you will be doing your best to help with the recovery. If there are difficult questions that you do not know the answer to such as, "Is Dad going to die?" answer with "I don't know, but he is receiving the best medical care and doing all that he can to get better."

- Share some of your own concerns and feelings about what has happened. Children respond well when you model for them that talking openly about feelings is okay. Convey to them a sense of hope and confidence that the family will work together to get through this difficult time.

- Explain to the children, especially as rehabilitation progresses, some of the lifestyle changes that will be occurring. If there is going to be a change in roles such that the sick parent may be doing fewer or different jobs around the house, inform them. If you will be expecting more responsibility from your older children, even temporarily, discuss it with them and ask for their input. However, be careful about giving them too much responsibility that takes away from their normal childhood. Involve your children in some of the planning of how things will be different in the house and in their lives.

- If there will be changes in the way the family eats and what types of food will be kept in the house, talk with your children as time progresses to see how they feel about this. The ideal situation is when the whole family makes lifestyle changes together. However, you may be more likely to find that compromises, especially with growing children who have variable nutritional needs and tastes, are more acceptable to everyone.

- If you suspect your children are having more serious problems coping, seek professional help from a psychologist or school counselor. Inform your children's teachers so that they may pay closer attention to your children's needs.

- Finally, reassure your children that they had nothing to do with the heart attack. Children have a way of sometimes blaming themselves for bad occurrences, and they need reassurance that the heart attack was not their fault, even if there may have been some arguing or disagreeing with the sick parent. Remind them that they do not have to take care of you or the sick parent but that the whole family will be taking care of each other.

When You Are the Child

If you are an adult child of a parent who has suffered a heart attack, you may be feeling fear, worry, guilt, anger, and so on. You may also suddenly find yourself in the role of having to take care of your sick parent. This, in addition to your own responsibilities, can be overwhelming. Be sure to not align yourself with your healthy parent in order to shield your sick parent from stress or in sympathy of all the changes that the healthy parent must endure. For example, don't exclude your sick parent from important discussions and decisions in order to protect him or her. This will be stressful for you and, in the long run, strain family relationships. In turn, do not take sides with your sick parent, who may be complaining about the other not doing enough. While this is often easier said than done, try to remain neutral and lovingly encourage your parents to talk to each other about their fears and concerns.

Try to stay connected to your parents in a loving manner while at the same time not neglecting your own family if you have one. This is often difficult, especially when you have assumed responsibility to take care of your sick parent physically, as well as emotionally. Ask for assistance and get support for yourself as needed instead of trying to be superhuman. Even if you are the only available caregiver, you can still consider part-time assistance from home health care agencies, or you can ask close friends for simple things like running an errand. Your local cardiac rehabilitation program can refer you to additional forms of assistance.

Finally, remember that you did not do anything to cause the heart attack—there are always multiple factors. And overworking yourself by trying to take care of everything for your sick parent will not necessarily prevent the occurrence of another one. Try to resolve any long-standing conflict with your sick parent so that you can have a close and supportive relationship. It will be the best thing you can do for your parent and for yourself.

6

Sex after a Heart Attack

Once you feel more secure in the idea that you will survive your heart attack, fears other than those about death may overwhelm you. Concerns about being able to live the way you used to are common. These include anxieties about your sexual life. You may recall stories you've heard about people dropping dead of heart attacks during sex, and you may feel you might as well give up on that part of your life altogether. If your partner has had a heart attack, you may avoid discussion of sex and the whole issue in general, due to your own fears that sex may be dangerous for him or her. Studies suggest that the frequency of sexual activities decreases in a substantial 40 to 70 percent of persons after having a heart attack, CABG, or stroke (Schover and Jensen 1988).

Do not despair, however, because these people may be depriving themselves needlessly. Studies recently done indicate that engaging in sexual activity is not likely to trigger a heart attack—even if you have heart disease or have had a prior heart attack (DeBusk 1996; Muller et al. 1996). Though sexual activity *slightly* increases chances of heart attack in the average person, this risk is so small that it is not really of practical significance. For instance, your risk appears to go from one in a million per hour to two in a million per hour in the two hours after having sex. And the risk increases for only that immediate period surrounding sex. After two hours, this increased risk disappears. Also, if you have had a heart attack or other form of heart disease, your risks for heart attack during sex don't appear to be any greater than those of a healthy person.

And there's even better news: if you exercise regularly, there is no increased risk of heart attack after sexual activity. The news is not as good if you tend to live a sedentary life. Your risks for triggering a heart attack during sex—or during any other kind of physically strenuous activity—are greater if you are sedentary. Regular physical exercise, at least two to three times per week, appears to protect against heart disease and reduce risks associated with engaging in any strenuous physical activities—including sex. When well-conditioned, your heart rate does not increase as much during heavy exercise as it does when it has not been conditioned. In the words of David Sobel and Robert Ornstein (1996), if you are physically fit, then you can "put your heart into sexual activity without unduly taxing it."

Although it appears that sex is generally a safe endeavor, there are certain situations in which you increase your risks. The majority of heart attacks that happen after sex occur in an unfamiliar place and with an unfamiliar partner. Dr. Eduardo Chapunoff, in his book *Sex and the Cardiac Patient* (1991), discusses how extramarital affairs may increase strain on your heart. The following aspects of extramarital activities may increase your risk:

- Higher levels of emotional stress due to guilt, fear of being discovered, or having to rush due to time constraints

- Attempts to please a new partner or prove sexual potency by engaging in physically challenging activities that are outside the typical range of behaviors

- Greater tendency to ignore symptoms of angina triggered by sexual activity and neglecting taking nitroglycerin or taking breaks due to pride, embarrassment, or wanting to impress a new partner

- Greater tendency to overindulge in food or alcohol or both— all of which increase strain on the heart, especially when closely followed by the physical exertion of sex

It appears that extramarital involvement can literally be a heart-breaking affair.

Discussion with Your Doctor

Your doctor should be the one to initiate a discussion about sex after a heart attack. However, this is not always the case. Many doctors avoid or neglect doing this, perhaps due to discomfort in discussing the area of sexuality. Additionally, many doctors have not been formally trained in how to deal with this important issue. Sometimes, physicians focus exclusively on the physical recovery of your heart and body to the neglect of issues pertaining to your lifestyle.

Whatever the reasons, a lack of attention to this area can be detrimental. You may mistakenly assume that if your doctor doesn't bring it up, then this means that sex is either not an important issue for you or that you won't be able to, or shouldn't, resume a healthy sex life. If your doctor does not include sexuality when discussing your recovery from a heart attack, then it will be up to you to ask. Here are sample questions you can use to guide your discussion with your doctor:

- How will my heart condition and my heart medications affect my sex life?
- When can I resume sexual activities with my partner?
- Are there any sexual activities or positions I should avoid?
- When should I take my medications (in relation to timing for sexual activities)?
- What should I do if I have chest pains, or other symptoms, during sex?
- I have problems with (choose one or more of the following). What does this mean and what can I do about it?

  _____ Pain during sex

  _____ Low or no sexual desire

  _____ Pain with erections

  _____ Pain during ejaculation

  _____ Becoming physically aroused

  _____ Soft erections

  _____ Premature ejaculation

  _____ No erection

  _____ Achieving orgasms

- I had problems with (choose one or more of the above) even before my heart attack. What does this mean and what can I do about it?
- Can you suggest a professional I can see to offer help with sexual counseling?

When to Resume Sex after a Heart Attack

When you can resume sexual activities depends on a number of factors, including the condition of your heart, your general medical condition, psychological state, your own and your partner's functioning, and your relationship with your partner. Talk with your doctor about specific recommendations for you.

Issues That Affect Your Sex Drive

Generally speaking, if your recovery from the heart attack has been uncomplicated, you may be able to resume sexual activities within a few weeks. However, sex is not a straightforward physical process. Issues like your psychological state and relationship with your partner must be considered. For example, concerns about your ability to perform sexually—sometimes called performance anxiety—can make you avoid sexual interactions and interfere with your performance when you do get around to trying sex again. If your mind is preoccupied with fears about your performance, you won't be able to enjoy the experience as much. If these anxieties are persistent, you will also be more likely to have difficulties like impotence or problems achieving orgasm, because anxiety distracts you from focusing on the pleasurable side of sex.

Fears of having a heart attack during sex can hopefully be put to rest by knowledge of the facts, as discussed earlier. This is tricky, however, because normal signs of sexual arousal, such as increased heart rate, blood pressure, and sweating, may be misinterpreted as cardiac symptoms. You can be reassured by the fact that sexual activity leads to only moderate increases in heart rate and blood pressure, and these levels tend to return to normal within about two minutes after orgasm. Studies suggest that the actual cardiac demands of sexual activities and orgasm are similar to the demands of a mildly stressful work situation or climbing a flight of stairs (Bohlen et al. 1984; Tardif 1989).

Depression, a common response to a heart attack, is another factor that often leads to low sexual desire and sexual difficulties.

Sexual difficulties, or dysfunctions, include problems in one or more of the stages of sexual responsiveness. In women, difficulties may include low sex drive, lack of physical arousal (less moisture or lubrication in the vagina), pain during intercourse, or problems achieving orgasm. Men may also experience low sexual desire as well as problems achieving erections, premature ejaculation, inability to ejaculate, or pain during intercourse.

If you or your partner have one or more of these problems, talk with your doctor about potential causes. The same kinds of difficulties that contribute to heart disease may also lead to sexual problems. Factors like diabetes, high blood pressure, smoking, or alcohol abuse may contribute to sexual problems. For example, atherosclerosis can interfere with blood flow to other body areas, including the pelvic region. Because erections depend on blood flow to the penis, atherosclerosis in this area can lead to problems with getting an erection.

Some cardiac medications have sexual side effects. Other drugs that can affect your sexual performance include sedatives (including alcohol), antidepressants, and some pain medications (such as narcotics). If you think your medications may be interfering with your sex life, talk with your doctor. Never stop taking or adjust doses of your medications without first speaking with your physician. There are often alternate medications that can be substituted and have fewer sexual side effects.

Fatigue or pain associated with heart disease may lessen sexual desire and enjoyment. Additionally, your sexual self-image depends on how attractive you feel physically and how capable you feel in satisfying your partner's needs. If you feel damaged or less attractive as a person because of your medical condition, then your self-esteem and ability to enjoy sex can suffer. If you have had a CABG, for instance, you may feel self-conscious about the scarring on your chest and leg. Women are especially vulnerable to anxieties about their body image. Rather than avoiding sexual contact and intimacy because of this, however, you can make some adjustments that enhance your comfort and confidence levels. For example, if you are a woman who has had a CABG, consider wearing romantic lingerie to conceal the scars until you feel more comfortable with them.

Marital or relationship conflicts may also adversely affect your sex life. Partners who are fearful that sex may trigger a heart attack may avoid the topic. This avoidance may be misinterpreted as rejection, leading to further loss of self-esteem and concerns about sexual activities. As a partner of someone with heart disease, ask if you can be involved in a cardiac rehabilitation program with your partner. There, you can get important information about your partner's physical capabilities. For example, witnessing a stress EKG can reassure you about what kind of physical exertion is safe for your partner. This kind of involvement can make you, as a couple, more likely to resume a better intimate life. Chronic tension or unhappiness in relationships not only leads to an unsatisfying sex life, but it's also a strain on your heart. Psychological counseling or marital counseling may be needed before sexual issues can be addressed.

How to Approach Sex after a Heart Attack

Before you resume sexual activities after a heart attack, it's important to examine your beliefs about sexuality in general. Sexuality is one of those areas clouded by myths and misconceptions. Some of these myths are particularly damaging to older people or to those who've had a serious medical problem. Your beliefs can interfere with your sexual adjustment by preventing you from gaining new skills and attitudes. Challenge your beliefs by considering the following myths and facts:

Myths

- Sex is only for the young and beautiful. Older people can't enjoy sex.
- Lovemaking must involve intercourse.
- Lovemaking must lead to orgasm.
- Sex saps your strength and therefore is harmful to those not in perfect health.
- Too much sex is unhealthy.
- Engaging in masturbation (self-stimulation) is dirty, or only for those hard-up individuals who can't get a partner.

Facts

- Though changes in your sexual reactions occur with age, sexual interest and activity are common for people in their sixties and seventies, and often beyond.
- Lovemaking includes a range of activities, not all of which include intercourse. Hugging, cuddling, kissing, caressing, and body massage are important expressions of intimacy that do not include a focus on orgasm or intercourse. Petting and caressing of erogenous areas (genitals and breasts) may be done with or without a focus on orgasm.
- Sexual activity can provide a healthy workout for your heart. During vigorous exercise associated with sex, you can burn four or five calories per minute. This is roughly equivalent to dancing, hiking, or playing tennis. Not only does sex feel good, but it can also reduce a sense of isolation, improve your relationship with your partner, and strengthen a sense of intimacy—as well as your heart health.
- Masturbating usually begins in childhood and continues throughout life in both sexes and in people with or without a regular sexual partner. It is not dirty or deviant, but is common, natural, and a healthy part of sexual activities.

After reading these myths and facts, try challenging any incorrect beliefs you have. If left alone, they could stand in the way of a better sex life for you and your partner. The following suggestions will help ease your sexual adjustment after your heart attack and improve your sex life in general.

Communicate

Talk with your partner openly about your feelings, fears of changes in your sexual responses, and worries about your health. Sharing feelings and concerns will make you both more relaxed and accepting.

Talk also about what is pleasurable for you and what is painful. If you've never talked about sex openly before, use this as an opportunity to share your desires, pleasures, likes, and dislikes more openly.

Take It Slowly

Resume lovemaking gradually by starting out with low-key but enjoyable activities, like cuddling, kissing, and caressing. One technique that has been used successfully to remove pressure associated with performance anxiety, and to enhance a focus on whole-body erotic feelings, is called *sensate focusing*. It involves sensual kinds of touching that allow you to improve your ability to give and receive pleasure in a gradual, relaxed progression. Here's how to go about it:

1. Agree to begin by having a ban on intercourse. The focus initially will be on touching and caressing each other without anticipating or worrying about sexual performance or intercourse.

2. Set the mood. Make the atmosphere as erotic and romantic as possible by including candles, soft music, or other props you enjoy. Even though the focus is not on intercourse or orgasm, it should be on romance and sensuality.

3. Begin by lightly touching or massaging your partner's body, covering all the areas from head to toes, front and back. Experiment with different kinds of touch, using different parts of your body (for instance, your mouth or lips in addition to hands) to do the touching. This is not a typical back rub or body massage. Though you want to be relaxed, no one should be so relaxed that they fall asleep. Keep a focus on the sensual, erotic aspects of your touching.

4. Avoid touching genitals the first few times you do this. The goal is not arousal or orgasm, but to increase the pleasure and sharing that go along with whole-body touching and to enhance intimacy and closeness.

5. Keep talking to a minimum. The exception is sharing about what touches feel good or uncomfortable. Sharing sexual fantasies or memories of past rewarding experiences can also increase closeness and sensuality. After about fifteen to thirty minutes, switch places and have your partner touch you in a similar fashion.

6. During later interactions, gradually include caressing of genitals and breasts. But don't rush to include intercourse. It's better to take it slowly. With time, and when you feel ready, then let intercourse happen.

David Sobel and Robert Ornstein provide a wonderful description of these techniques and others in their book *The Healthy Mind,
Healthy Body Handbook* (1996). Additional ideas on sexual issues or
problems can be found in references listed in the appendix.

Experiment

If you're concerned and self-conscious about how your first sexual interaction will go after your heart attack, you can experiment
first with masturbation. If you're comfortable with this activity, it can
put some of your fears to rest and make the first experience with
your partner less anxiety-provoking.

After you progress to including intercourse among your sexual
interactions, be open to trying different positions. The missionary position, facing each other, with the male on top of the female, is the
most common position for intercourse. However, you may find other
positions more comfortable (or more stimulating and exciting). For
example, if you have heart failure, you may notice greater shortness
of breath when lying on your back. Men using the missionary position
can experience greater fatigue from supporting themselves on elbows
or hands and knees. As an alternative, the female-on-top position
may reduce this discomfort or strain. In addition, a side-by-side, face-
to-face—or a side-by-side, female back to male front—position can
avoid any weight-bearing burdens and lessen the strain of either partner supporting him- or herself.

Include a Range of Activities
as Lovemaking

Not all sexual encounters have to include intercourse. Spend
more time with affectionate touch, caressing, and cuddling, which do
not always lead to intercourse. These activities are less strenuous physically, enhance intimacy and closeness with your partner, and build
up sensual, erotic feelings without any pressure to perform.

Don't Rush In

Be cautious to not attempt sex prematurely. Some heart attack
survivors, most often men, become so worried or curious about how
their heart attack may affect sexual abilities that they test it out too
quickly. This can put unnecessary strain on the heart before it's had
time to heal.

Don't Procrastinate

On the other hand, don't wait too long either. Many heart attack survivors postpone sex due to erring on the side of caution and to fears of physical harm coming from this exertion. However, the longer you wait after your doctor has given you the go-ahead for sex, the more likely you are to be exceedingly nervous and to have difficulties with performance anxiety.

Summary: Tips on Resuming Sexual Activity after a Heart Attack

The following suggestions were adapted from recommendations of Dr. Eduardo Chapunoff in *Sex and the Cardiac Patient* (1991).

- Obtain your doctor's approval.

- Be watchful for cardiac symptoms that occur during sexual interactions. If you experience symptoms of angina, stop, rest, and take medications, like nitroglycerin, as prescribed by your doctor. Don't let pride prevent you from caring for your heart.

- As much as possible, prevent stress associated with sexual interactions. Allow adequate time without interruptions and prepare a relaxed atmosphere. Find the optimal time of day for lovemaking—when fatigue is at its lowest. Plan dates for intimacy so these arrangements can be made in advance.

- Avoid excessive physical demands. Every once in a while, have interactions that don't include intercourse. On taking it slowly, Dr. Robert Eliot suggests that you "ease up on the throttle and work on your technique" (Eliot and Breo 1984). Sexual gymnastics are not required for satisfying experiences. And don't rush— studies have shown that extended foreplay decreases cardiac stress associated with orgasm.

- Pay attention to the room temperature and ventilation. Cold temperatures can lead to decreased blood supply to the heart and chest discomfort. Hot temperatures can increase sweating, shortness of breath, and feeling weak or light-headed.

- Avoid sexual activity after heavy meals or consumption of alcohol. After eating, your heart has increased demands in pumping extra blood to your digestive system. Wait about three or four hours after a heavy meal before having sex. Excessive alcohol can lead to irregular heartbeats, especially when com- bined with physical exertion.

- Take medications correctly as prescribed by your doctor.

- Ask for help or advice from your doctor when you need it. If you notice changes in your angina symptoms or problems, such as greater fatigue, shortness of breath, feeling faint, or sleep difficulties after sex, call your doctor.

- Pay attention to your partner. Involve your spouse or partner in discussions with doctors and in cardiac rehabilitation, if possible. Openly communicate your needs, desires, and fears to your partner.

- Keep a sense of humor. Negative attitudes will only contribute to more failures. Be playful and light-hearted in sexual encounters. Couples who adjust best sexually are those who are playful, see lovemaking as including a range of activities, and are open and flexible in experimenting.

Generally speaking, if you had a good sex life prior to your heart attack, then you can most likely return to it after your recovery. And even if you had sexual problems before your attack, advice from your doctor and/or sexual counseling can be helpful in overcoming problems like impotence, premature ejaculation, loss of sexual desire, difficulties reaching orgasm, or painful sex. Even if your difficulties stem from a medical disorder or condition, there are treatments that can help restore sexual functioning. Don't minimize the importance of a healthy sexual life. It can lead to a positive sense of well-being, an improved intimate relationship, and a healthier heart.

PART 3

Lifestyle Management: Traditional Risk Factors

Patients should be interested not only in the years left in their lives, but also in the liveliness of their years.

—Robert F. DeBusk, M.D.

7

Motivation

We are now going to spend the remainder of the book talking about how *you* can change your risk factors for heart disease. *You* have control over the health of your heart.

Before we talk about the techniques and strategies for changing your lifestyle, let's look at motivation: without motivation and a commitment to the changes, information about strategies are just that—information.

What Motivates People to Change?

When presented with information about their health and the changes they need to make to their lifestyle, what *exactly* motivates people to make these changes? Well, the fear of death is a great motivator for change. Frequently, after patients suffer a heart attack, they begin to make changes in their life. For example, they may quit smoking and improve their diets. However, it's also not uncommon for people to lose their motivation to continue these changes. They may return to smoking or gradually return to their poor eating habits. Does this sound familiar?

Are there certain factors that help people stay committed to the changes they make? There are twenty-one commonly studied theories and models that explain how certain feelings and beliefs can contribute to healthy behaviors. For the purposes of this book, we won't review all of the research on these theories. However, to give you an idea of how much research has been conducted simply on what motivates us, between 1992 and 1994 there were about five hundred scientific articles published on this topic!

The following basic themes and concepts of these theories will help you identify what motivates you and how you can stay committed to healthy behaviors.

Perceived Threat

This concept refers to whether or not you believe you're going to get sick in the first place and if you accept your diagnosis of heart disease. That is, what are your beliefs about your own susceptibility to developing heart disease or of making the disease worse? Also, it refers to how serious you believe your condition to be. For example, do you tend to deny the seriousness of your illness and the impact that your continued risky behavior can have on a future heart attack? Read the following statements and decide if you strongly agree, agree, disagree, or strongly disagree with each one:

1. Cigarette smoking can cause heart disease. _____

2. My cigarette smoking will cause heart disease. _____

3. My cigarette smoking will lead to another heart attack. _____

4. High cholesterol levels are harmful to the heart. _____

5. If I continue to cheat on my diet, I will significantly increase my chances for another heart attack. _____

If you answered "Agree" to statement 1, but disagree with statements 2 and 3, you may generally feel that smoking is harmful, but not perceive it as enough of a threat to change your behavior. In contrast, if you believe that you're at risk for developing a disease and that the likelihood of it occurring is high, you'll be more motivated to engage in healthy behaviors. Use the following strategies for more realistically evaluating your susceptibility to disease and future heart attacks:

- **Obtain accurate and specific information from your doctor.** Often patients will claim that the doctor never specifically said that their smoking or their diet can cause damage to their heart. This miscommunication may be due in part to the patients *not asking direct questions* because then they can assume if it wasn't directly stated, than it must not be that serious. Isn't the unconscious mind a great thing? It allows us to deny and distort information as we choose. In addition, doctors often make assumptions that some things are so obvious they go without saying, like "Smoking is dangerous to your heart." However, although you may know intellectually that smoking, a high-fat diet, and lack of exercise are dangerous to your heart without a doctor directly pointing it out, it doesn't carry the same weight as a doctor's warning. Therefore, be prepared to ask your doctor specific questions about your risk factors and your heart disease, even if you aren't sure you want to hear the answers.

- **Objectively evaluate the information you are given about changes in your lifestyle.** We are often very comfortable with giving advice to other people we care about. We can easily say, "You really shouldn't smoke," or "I'm concerned about your weight and the stress it's placing on your heart," or "You seem depressed and it's affecting your health." However, when it comes to ourselves that advice is often lost. Although you may be able to say, "I really shouldn't eat this" or "I really should be exercising," you may also follow it up with excuses that give you permission to continue with the behavior. For example, you may say to yourself, "I really shouldn't eat this bacon and egg breakfast but this one time won't hurt me" or "I know I should exercise on a regular basis but I'm a busy person, always running around, and therefore I get a lot of exercise." If you could step outside of yourself for a moment and listen to what you're saying to yourself, you would probably be able to come back with an attack on those excuses. Would you allow a friend or loved one to continue to eat a diet high in fat with the knowledge that he or she could very likely suffer another heart attack? What would you say to them? Can you say those things to yourself? Why shouldn't you say those things to yourself?

- **Pay attention to signals and messages from your body.** How many times have you experienced a symptom such as shortness of breath, tightness in your chest, or fatigue that you dismissed as indigestion or stress and did nothing about it? Do you tend to minimize or ignore symptoms in your body? It is important to tune in to what your body is saying even if you're afraid or worried about what it may mean. Ignoring it will not make it go away and it will not make the consequences any less real. On the contrary, ignoring messages, symptoms, or signals from your body can lead to serious complications or death. Therefore, it's important to risk possibly feeling foolish that it may be nothing or facing your worst fear, which is that it is indeed something. Either way, it's important to let your body guide you. If the worst thing that happens is that you feel foolish for worrying over indigestion, and the best thing is that you save your life, take the risk. Don't ignore any symptoms.

Beliefs about Immediate Benefits

We are unlikely to change our behavior unless we believe that there will be an immediate benefit to our health. Telling someone to monitor the amount of saturated fats in their diet when they are not currently experiencing cardiac symptoms is unlikely to be successful. Similarly, telling a smoker that she needs to quit smoking to reduce her risk for having a heart attack is not as motivating as telling her that the amount of nicotine found in her cervical mucous during a routine pap smear leaves her two to three times more likely to develop cervical cancer than a woman who doesn't smoke. This kind of information is immediate and subsequently tends to motivate us to make active changes as we envision the immediate benefit to our health. Here are some techniques that may help you recognize and stay focused on immediate benefits:

- **Visualize yourself benefiting from the changes.** For example, instead of feeling deprived, try visualizing benefits to your heart as you learn to eat less food with saturated fats. As you eat, actually turn on the camera in your head and observe the effects that the food is having on your arteries. See them free and open and readily allowing blood to flow without the clogging effect of cholesterol and fat. See your heart pumping at a regular and comfortable rate without having to work so hard. Make this a conscious process when you are eating.

- **Remind yourself that you are making the right choice.** For example, tell yourself as you exercise that you are lowering your cholesterol, keeping your weight down, and improving the overall functioning of your heart. Pay attention to the feeling of your heart beating during exercise, regular and strong. Know that you are working hard to keep your heart healthy and your mind strong.

- **Gather information about risks for future heart attacks and what you can do to prevent it.** Knowledge is power, so don't run from it. Actively seek it out and remind yourself that you have the power to make changes. You are not powerless over your disease. Many times cardiac patients feel helpless and therefore minimize any immediate benefits that their behavior may have over their heart disease. They often feel that if they dismiss the importance of making changes, then they don't have to try and potentially set themselves up to fail. Have you ever said that to yourself? Do you objectively look at the information about the immediate benefits to your heart that you can achieve by making lifestyle changes? Or do you deny and ignore the information because you are afraid of failing and therefore believe that it would be better not to commit to making the changes in the first place? Examine your beliefs and thoughts about the immediate and well-documented facts about how diet, exercise, smoking cessation and other lifestyle changes can have on the health of your heart. What do you say to yourself about this information? How do you set yourself up to fail? What convinces and motivates you to see and believe these benefits?

Beliefs about the Cost of Making a Change

When we are confronted with information about our health and the changes we need to make, a couple of thoughts usually come to mind. First, we begin to weigh the benefit of making a change and the price we will pay. For example, you might weigh the benefits of eating a healthy diet versus the loss of eating whatever you want. Look at the following two examples of a cost-benefit analysis.

Benefits to a Healthy Diet

• Improve my heart disease

• Improve my energy

• Keep my weight down

Cost of Changing My Diet

• More effort in reading labels

• More time initially in meal preparation

• Reduce my risk of having another heart attack

Benefits to a Healthy Diet

• Marginally improve my heart disease

• Keep weight down

Cost of Changing My Diet

• Deprive myself of the foods I enjoy

• Need a degree in how to read labels

• An inconvenience to my family to have to watch what we eat

• Social life will be altered by where we can eat out

In the first example, it's clear that the benefits to changing the diet significantly outweigh the costs. Not only are there *more* benefits listed, but the kind of benefits are significant. Improving heart disease, avoiding another heart attack, and improving energy, which makes life more pleasurable, are clearly valued by this person. Even the costs that are associated with this change are viewed as minor in comparison to the benefits. That is, this person is probably thinking, "I may need to initially spend a little more time preparing meals and learning to read food labels, but in return I may save my life."

In contrast, the other example demonstrates that the cost of changing this person's diet is too high for the perceived small benefit. Notice the language: "deprive myself," "inconvenience to my family," and "marginally improve my heart disease."

How do you view changes that you need to make in your life to improve your health? Try to do a cost-benefit analysis for yourself. Notice the language you use and the actual number of items on each side of the analysis. If you're going to make changes, you need to honestly assess how *real* you believe the health threat is for you and

what cost you perceive yourself having to pay for what kind of benefit. Be honest. Even if you find that intellectually you know what
you are supposed to be saying, what do you *really* believe? Once you
have evaluated your beliefs about benefits and costs, you will be in
a better position to improve your beliefs about the benefits by obtaining more accurate information, using incentives, or getting more
reassurance.

Self-Confidence

Do you listen to a health message and find yourself acknow-
ledging that while it makes sense, deep inside you're thinking, "I
could never really do that"? As you're reading through this book,
are you saying to yourself, "I don't believe I could actually make
those changes in my life," "There are too many changes," or "I'm
not committed enough to keep up with the changes"? These statements are a reflection of your self-confidence. Self-confidence involves
a commitment to the healthy behavior and a belief in your own ability
to stick with that commitment. How confident are you that you can
tolerate high-risk situations without relapsing into unhealthy behavior? High-risk situations usually involve times when you are around
others and having a good time, or when you're feeling depressed,
angry, or anxious. It can also include situations when you are craving
something. This could be a cigarette, salty foods, alcohol, and so on.
To more clearly evaluate the strength of your confidence, read the
following statements and decide if you strongly agree, agree, disagree,
or strongly disagree:

1. I believe I can resist a cigarette when I'm feeling anxious.

2. I believe I can say no to foods high in fat when dining with
   friends in a restaurant.

3. I believe I can resist the temptation for sweets when I'm depressed.

4. I believe I'll continue to exercise when I feel angry at myself
   and others.

5. I believe I can resist a cigarette when I'm at a party with
   other smokers.

6. I believe I can change my hectic, fast-paced style of living,
   even if my spouse or business partners do not.

7. I believe I can learn to effectively use stress reduction techniques.

8. I believe I can learn better time management techniques for
   when I'm under stress.

9. I believe I have the ability to continue a regular exercise program even if others around me do not support exercise.

10. I believe I can learn to shop and cook in a more heart-healthy way even when my time is limited.

How confident are you in your ability to make healthy changes? Did you strongly agree with the majority of questions? Which situations or feelings did you feel least confident in resisting temptation? For example, if you answered disagree or strongly disagree to questions that involved making changes when around others or when depressed, then these are your high-risk situations. It's important to note what these situations are so that you may better prepare for them. Confidence is built when we are able to have several small measures of success in high-risk situations. So if you notice that resisting high-fat foods is particularly difficult for you when you're dining out with friends, then small improvements will be felt as successes to be built upon. If each time you go out you make one small healthy change in your food selection, then you'll improve your confidence in making even more subsequent changes the next time that you go out. This will improve your confidence and commitment to sticking with your healthy behavior.

Self-Image

Another important part of staying committed to healthy behaviors is how you view yourself. When you look at yourself do you see what you want to? In your mind, do you envision a healthy, active person, but when you look in the mirror do you see a "couch potato"?

The image we have of ourselves comes from inside. This is our self-image. The image can either be quite distorted or realistic—or a combination of both. Consider the following scenario:

Joe is a fifty-year-old upper middle class businessman who has always succeeded in life. After Joe's angioplasty procedure and prior to his first heart attack, he was asked to describe himself. He called himself a healthy and active person. On further examination about what Joe actually meant by healthy and active, we asked him to provide a list of descriptions about a healthy and active person. The following is Joe's list of descriptors for a healthy and active person.

- Busy and on the go
- Achievement-oriented
- Driven to succeed
- Not lazy
- Happy

- Energetic

- Pays careful attention to never skipping meals

- Doesn't smoke

Since Joe originally described himself as a healthy and active person, much of his self-image is included in his list of descriptions. However, on closer inspection with Joe it became clear that his image was distorted and based on inaccurate information. Specifically, Joe stated that he was always busy and on the go, energized, and not lazy. However, what Joe neglected to see was that he was busy burning up energy with a fast-paced lifestyle that was leaving him chronically stressed and fatigued. His stress was managed by aggressively interacting with his staff at work and placing unusually high demands on his family.

He believed that he was healthy because he felt he was getting ample exercise by always "running here and there." However, the reality was that Joe was not getting exercise—he was getting more stressed. Constant motion and activity is not the same as healthy exercise.

When we interviewed Joe, he also took pride in his commitment to never skip meals. Again on closer examination, although Joe was able to outline some healthy choices in his diet, his usual business lunches and dinners consisted of high-fat foods and alcohol that were usually consumed in a hurried manner. His response regarding the reality of his diet was, "Well, I eat healthy foods when I'm home with my family for dinner." This actually consisted of only three evenings a week and the weekends. Joe admitted that when he was with business colleagues he felt uncomfortable and mildly embarrassed about ordering healthy meals while others were eating steak and potatoes with sour cream and butter. He didn't want to feel like an outsider or, worse, a "sick person." His dietary choices, along with his relatively high consumption of alcohol, made him feel "healthy, normal, and part of the group."

Joe's image of himself as healthy and active was in part generated from his belief that if you get up early in the morning, run all day long, are productive and accomplish tasks, eat three meals a day, get adequate sleep, and are not experiencing any "real" physical symptoms, then you must be healthy.

Unfortunately for Joe, the realization that this belief was inaccurate and his image of himself was distorted only came to him after he suffered a heart attack. It was at this point that we began to work with Joe on developing a more accurate image of himself as a healthy and active person. The following strategies were used:

- **Clarify your values.** Joe began to see that all of his self-esteem came from his accomplishments at work. So, he made changes at home that helped him focus on his personal values. He became more involved with his children's activities and events. Through this reengagement with the family, Joe discovered that he took pride in being a father to his children. He recognized that his self-worth did not only come from work, but could also come from the other roles he played in his life, like father and husband. Joe continued to be achievement-oriented and constantly strived to accomplish business goals, but he was better able to find a balance in his life.

- **Find healthy role models.** One of the big hang-ups for Joe was feeling that he didn't fit in with his colleagues when he tried to make changes to his lifestyle. He felt awkward ordering different food in the restaurant, reducing his alcohol consumption, and managing his temper in a different way. He felt that others would view him as ineffective and somehow "sick." An important strategy was for Joe to find healthy role models. Through some networking, Joe was able to connect with other executives who had adopted a new lifestyle for better health. Some had heart disease, some, like Joe, had suffered a heart attack, and some were simply trying to reduce their risk for heart disease. Joe began to see that you could still be successful, motivated, and hardworking, but in a more balanced fashion. Three times a week, Joe would meet other colleagues at the gym during lunch hour to exercise, and the other two days he'd meet with his old colleagues for lunch. He soon began to feel more confident in ordering healthier lunches.

- **Imagine yourself as a healthy person.** Joe's initial image of himself was quite distorted and based on false beliefs. With a newfound insight into his false image, he began to more accurately see himself in his mind's eye. He spent a portion of his morning before launching into his busy routine to imagine his "new self." He made positive statements to himself about the changes he'd begun to make and how much better the health of his heart had become. He continued to imagine his heart beating stronger and more comfortably. While imagining this improved self, he reminded himself about the benefits of these changes, such as having a longer and happier life with his family and friends while continuing to succeed and excel in his professional life. He now had a different image of a healthy and active person.

Can you relate to Joe's story? What do you share in common with him? Take a few minutes to describe your image of yourself. How accurate is it? Would others agree with your view? More fully understanding the image you have of yourself will help spark and sustain your motivation for healthy changes.

Environmental Cues

Many of the motivating factors we've talked about so far involve changes that you need to make inside yourself. There are also environmental changes you can make to support your efforts to change your unhealthy behaviors. Surrounding yourself with cues to remind you of your commitment to change and help you sustain changes can be quite useful. These may include

- Surrounding yourself with supportive people who share your commitment to a healthy lifestyle.

- Keeping healthy foods readily available to you. If you're hungry and in a hurry and there are no easy and healthy choices around, you're more likely to grab something quick and less healthy. It's just as easy to eat a bag of potato chips as it is to eat a bag of air-popped popcorn without butter or salt. The difference is if the chips are readily available to you in the cupboard and the popcorn seems like a hassle to make or get, you're more likely to make an unhealthy choice. Therefore, it's important to keep healthy and easy-to-prepare foods on hand.

- Having an exercise partner you work out with on a regular basis. This can serve as a cue to exercise. For example, it is Tuesday night and Sue is waiting for you at the gym. Tuesday night and Sue are cues or triggers for your exercise routine.

- Not having ashtrays or stray cigarettes around. This can serve as a reminder that you don't smoke and you are not encouraging others around you to smoke.

- Posting reminder notes for yourself that support your efforts to manage anger and frustration better. Your notes can remind you of the negative impact that anger has on your heart, or they can reinforce the improvement that your new style of anger management has had on your relationships.

- Keeping a list of your priorities and the amount of time committed to each task as a reminder of your improved time management techniques.

As you proceed with the next chapters, keep this information about motivation in your mind. Pay attention to those situations and behaviors where you feel your motivation and commitment may decrease. Return to this section as you learn specific techniques and strategies for keeping your risk factors for heart disease low and your quality of life better. Use this section to keep your mind open to the information and your motivation high.

8

Changing Your Diet

Of all the risk factors that have been associated with the development of heart disease, perhaps the most undisputed is being overweight and/or having high cholesterol from eating a diet high in fats. While it is one of the risk factors over which you have some control it is also one that may involve the biggest overall lifestyle change—changing what and how you eat on a daily basis. We are bombarded every day with messages and vivid images on TV and in magazines of delicious, mouthwatering food that is, more often than not, high in fat, cholesterol, and calories. Some of your favorite foods might be the very ones that are the most unhealthy for your heart. If your eating habits have included rich, fatty foods, then changing this risk factor will require a strong commitment from you and support from those around you. If your diet has been fairly healthy, then you will have an easier time making the necessary adjustments. Eating a heart-healthy diet will be the most important change you make for yourself.

Getting started changing any long-standing pattern is a daunting task. Changing what you eat is no exception, especially since it involves such a basic human function. You can approach this task by breaking it down into phases, gradually moving yourself to a new way of eating without having to make a drastic change all at once. The first step is to educate yourself about the impact of cholesterol, fats, and excess weight on your heart.

Cholesterol

The whole issue of cholesterol can be very confusing. You've been hearing about the dangers of cholesterol for years from your doctors and through the media. Product manufacturers go to great lengths to label and promote their product based on cholesterol information.

For most people, the very word *cholesterol* conjures up an image of something bad that should be avoided. Then, just as they begin to understand that concept, they hear about something called "good" cholesterol. What is "good" and "bad" cholesterol? Where does cholesterol come from? Which foods should be avoided and which foods should be included in your diet to control cholesterol? What role does exercise play in the reduction of cholesterol?

Take the following quiz to assess your current knowledge about cholesterol.

Cholesterol Quiz

1. What is cholesterol?
   a. Odorless, white, fatlike substance present in every cell in the body
   b. Fat found in certain foods
   c. White, sticky substance found on the surface of teeth

2. Cholesterol is bad for your health.
   a. True
   b. False

3. Cholesterol found in your body comes from
   a. The liver
   b. The liver and your diet
   c. The kidney and liver
   d. Plants and vegetables

4. Cholesterol levels for adults should ideally be below
   a. 300 mg/dl
   b. 200 mg/dl
   c. 20 mg/dl
   d. 30 mg/dl

5. High blood-cholesterol level is a major risk factor for
   a. Nose bleeds
   b. Coronary heart disease
   c. Prostate cancer
   d. Depression

6. What is HDL cholesterol?
   a. Good cholesterol that prevents the buildup of cholesterol in the arteries
   b. Bad cholesterol that causes the buildup of cholesterol in the arteries
   c. An artificial sweetener
   d. An advertising scam

7. What is LDL cholesterol?
   a. Bad cholesterol found only in the blood
   b. Good cholesterol found only in the blood
   c. Bad cholesterol found in fatty foods
   d. Good cholesterol found in spinach

8. Saturated fatty acids in foods
   a. Are a healthy source of vitamin C
   b. Lower blood cholesterol levels
   c. Raise blood cholesterol levels

9. _____ are primary sources of saturated fats.
   a. Vegetables
   b. Meats, poultry, and dairy products
   c. Candies, cookies, and soda pop

10. It is recommended that you eat less than _____ milligrams of cholesterol per day.
   a. 500
   b. 5000
   c. 300
   d. 3000

11. It is important to replace saturated fats with unsaturated fats such as polyunsaturated or monounsaturated fats because they help lower blood cholesterol.
   a. True
   b. False

12. _____ is a good source of polyunsaturated fatty acids.
   a. Chocolate
   b. Vegetable oil, such as sunflower, corn, and soybean
   c. Camphor oil

13. Soft margarines that come in tubs are better than hard sticks.
   a. True
   b. False

14. Aerobic exercise, such as bicycling or running, increases the level of HDL cholesterol and thereby reduces your risk for cardiovascular disease.
   a. True
   b. False

15. Overweight people tend to have higher cholesterol levels.
   a. True

b. False

16. Eating oat bran cereal (like oatmeal) can help to lower blood cholesterol.
   a. True
   b. False

Cholesterol Quiz Answers

1. What is cholesterol?
   a. It is an odorless, white, fatlike substance. Liver cells manufacture most of the cholesterol in your body.

2. Cholesterol is bad for your health.
   b. False. Cholesterol is necessary for the body to ensure proper functioning of the nervous system and certain cell membranes.

3. Cholesterol found in your body comes from
   b. Your liver manufactures a large percentage of the cholesterol in your body, and a high-fat diet increases the cholesterol in your blood.

4. Cholesterol levels for adults should ideally be below
   b. The National Cholesterol Education Panel (1987) classified levels of cholesterol. A blood cholesterol level below 200 mg/dl puts you at a lower risk for heart disease.

5. High blood-cholesterol level is a major risk factor for
   b. Coronary heart disease.

6. What is HDL cholesterol?
   a. HDL cholesterol can be thought of as the "H"ealthy cholesterol that prevents cholesterol from building up in the arteries and subsequently decreases chances for heart disease.

7. What is LDL cholesterol?
   a. LDL cholesterol, or "L"ousy cholesterol, is found only in the blood. It acts as a carrier for the cholesterol and fat in the blood. Having elevated levels of LDL is a significant risk factor for heart disease.

8. Saturated fatty acids in foods
   c. Increase cholesterol levels in the blood.

9. _____ are primary sources of saturated fats.
   b. Saturated fats can be found in meat, poultry skin, and dairy products (particularly eggs and most cheese). They can also be found in tropical oils such as palm and coconut oil.

10. It is recommended that you eat less than _____ milligrams of cholesterol per day.

    c. Cholesterol from your diet should be limited to under 300 mg/day.

11. It is important to replace saturated fats with unsaturated fats such as polyunsaturated or monounsaturated fats because they help lower blood cholesterol.

    a. True.

12. _____ is a good source of polyunsaturated fatty acids.

    b. Vegetable oil, such as sunflower, corn, and soybean, is a good source.

13. Soft margarines that come in tubs are better than hard sticks.

    a. True. Saturated fats are solid at room temperature. When a food has been hydrogenated, that means that hydrogen atoms have been added and the substance becomes solid.

14. Aerobic exercise, such as bicycling or running, increases the level of HDL cholesterol and thereby reduces your risk for cardiovascular disease.

    a. True. Aerobic exercise increases the HDL, which decreases risk for heart disease and helps to reduce total body fat, which then reduces levels of LDL (high levels of LDL are correlated with heart disease).

15. Overweight people tend to have higher cholesterol levels.

    a. True. A diet high in fat is also high in cholesterol.

16. Eating oat bran cereal can help to lower blood cholesterol.

    a. True. Foods that are high in soluble fibers, such as oat cereals, when added to a lowfat diet can reduce cholesterol by an additional 2 to 3 percent.

How did you do on the quiz? Were there things that surprised you about cholesterol? The one point that should be perfectly clear by now is that a high level of bad cholesterol is a major risk factor for cardiac disease. Therefore, keeping your total cholesterol level low is an important step in reducing your risk for the development or recurrence of cardiac disease. The first step to improving cholesterol levels is to understand the mechanisms of how cholesterol works in the body and to believe in the importance of keeping it low for your heart's sake.

Cholesterol is a substance that is necessary for our bodies to function. It is made in our bodies by the liver and in addition to being part of each cell membrane, it is used to make hormones such as estrogen, progesterone, and testosterone, essential for normal development in women and men. Cholesterol is also needed by the body to produce vitamin D and cortisol, a hormone used to fight infection and regulate blood sugar. In addition, it is used by the liver to help the body digest food that contains fat.

Cholesterol can also be found in all foods that come from animal sources. Foods such as vegetables, fruits, and grains do not contain cholesterol. When you get extra cholesterol from eating meat products, your body tries to balance this by adjusting the level of cholesterol it produces in the body and excreting any excess through the liver. There are two types of cholesterol, *high-density lipoprotein* (HDL) and *low-density lipoprotein* (LDL). *Lipoproteins* are substances that carry the cholesterol throughout the blood. LDLs carry cholesterol to the cells of your body for its functions, and HDLs carry excess cholesterol from the cells back to the liver for excretion. If most of the cholesterol in your blood is being carried by the HDLs out of the body through the liver, then there is less risk of it accumulating to dangerous levels in your body. However, if more of the cholesterol is carried by LDLs, then more cholesterol stays in your body. Hence, the popular terms, "bad" cholesterol for LDL and "good" cholesterol for HDL. You can remember this more easily by thinking of "L"ousy DL and "H"ealthy DL.

While it may appear that your body has its own mechanism for balancing cholesterol, this balance becomes disturbed if you con-sume too much cholesterol in your daily diet or have too much through heredity. Historically, our ancestors consumed much less cho-lesterol in their diets than we do today. Therefore, it's difficult for our bodies to handle all of the excess cholesterol contained in the modern diet of fatty meats, fast foods, and processed foods. After all, the body essentially makes almost all of the cholesterol that it needs by itself. The other factor that can upset your body's management of cholesterol is heredity or biological factors. Some people's bodies are not able to handle excess cholesterol in the blood as efficiently, thereby allowing it to accumulate.

High Cholesterol and Heart Disease

High cholesterol affects your heart in the following manner: When you consume too much cholesterol, the excess, carried by LDLs, can't be used by the body and begins to crowd in your blood. The LDLs begin to attach to the walls of your blood vessels and soon build into fatty *plaques*. This condition is known as *atherosclerosis*. The arteries then become narrowed, making it difficult for blood to flow smoothly. When the arteries of your heart become narrowed, blood flow to your heart is restricted and you can suffer chest pain. When blood flow to a part of your heart is completely cut off, the result is a heart attack.

To find out what your cholesterol level actually is, you need to have your health care provider perform standard cholesterol tests, which include testing total cholesterol, HDL, and LDL. Most experts agree that a total cholesterol level below 200 mg/dl is ideal. If your total cholesterol is higher, your LDL cholesterol level is high, and/or your HDL cholesterol level is low, there are several important things you can do to change these numbers and, ultimately, your risk for heart disease. A fourth number you'll see on your cholesterol profile is about your triglycerides. *Triglycerides* are fat molecules in your bloodstream that get transported to your cells for energy. A high level of triglycerides is also associated with coronary heart disease. See figure 8.1 for a breakdown of these numbers.

The Different Types of Fats

There are basically three types of fat that can be made: *saturated, polyunsaturated,* and *monounsaturated.* Foods that come from meat and dairy products contain saturated fats. They are solid at room temperature. Examples include butter, lard, the visible fat in meats, and the fat in milk (if the fat from milk is removed, it becomes solid at room temperature). Two vegetable fats that are high in saturated fats are coconut oil and palm oil. These two oils are used in foods such as nondairy creamers, baked goods, and candy. Cocoa butter, used in chocolates, is also high in saturated fats. *Polyunsaturated fats* are typically liquid at room temperature and are found in the seeds of some plants. Examples include oils made from corn, safflowers, sunflowers, cotton, and soybeans. *Monounsaturated fats,* also liquid at room temperature, are found in olive, canola, and rapeseed oil. When some of these oils are processed in order to be used for baking or to improve their shelf life, they become *hydrogenated* or *partially hydrogenated* and therefore more saturated. Examples of hydrogenated vegetable oils include margarine and vegetable shortening.

Saturated fats increase the levels of cholesterol in your blood. Polyunsaturated fats decrease levels of "bad" cholesterol (LDL) but can also decrease your "good" cholesterol, HDL, a little bit. Monounsaturated fats do even better by lowering your LDL cholesterol without lowering your HDL cholesterol. The more fat you consume in your diet, the more saturated fats and cholesterol will be causing damage to your heart. High calorie, high-fat diets are also typically high in cholesterol.

Modifying Your Diet

Now that you've read about the basics of cholesterol and its effects on your heart, the next step is to begin changing the amount of cholesterol and saturated fats that you consume every day. It can be

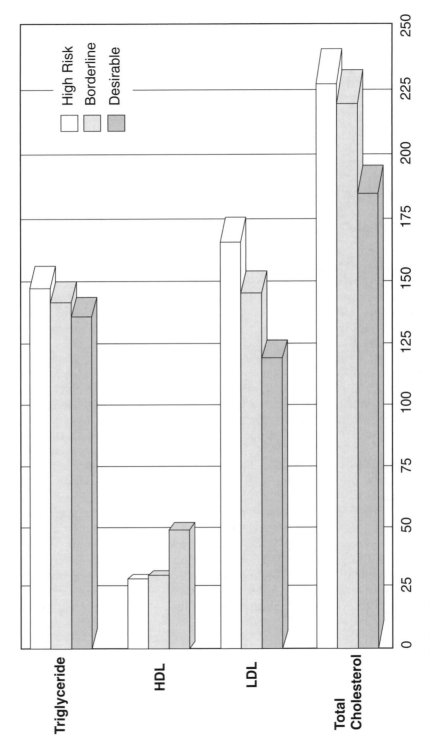

Figure 8.1   Cholesterol Numbers

difficult in the beginning to keep track of all of the information about amounts of cholesterol in each food and whether it is high in saturated fats or not. The recommended amount of cholesterol you should consume in your diet is less than 300 mg per day (the average person consumes about 400–500 mg per day). The American Heart Association recommends limiting your fat intake to no more than 30 percent of your daily calories and your saturated fat intake to less than 10 percent. Rather than focusing on the actual numbers, start by following these simple guidelines to keep your cholesterol levels and fat intake in a healthy range:

- **Limit your consumption of egg yolks.** One single egg yolk contains 250 mg of cholesterol! Limiting your consumption, then, is probably the single, quickest way of lowering your cholesterol. Remember that eggs are hidden in many foods you eat, like baked foods and processed foods. Try to eat no more than three egg yolks per week and instead substitute egg whites or egg substitute.

- **Try to avoid or reduce eating fatty meats and organ meats like liver.** Meats are high sources of saturated fats and cholesterol. Therefore, you should try to choose lean cuts of meat and eat smaller portions. *Prime cut* usually indicates a cut of meat that is higher in fat content. Meat that has a higher fat content may taste better, but the leaner meat, if prepared well, can also be moist and flavorful. Organ meats, like liver, contain a lot of cholesterol (270 mg for a three-ounce serving of liver). Table 8.1 lists some healthier choices of meat.

- **Reduce the amount of processed meat.** Foods such as hot dogs, bacon, bologna, and sausages contain too much fat.

- **Eat more chicken and less red meat.** Chicken has lower amounts of saturated fats, particularly when the skin is removed. Breast of chicken is a little healthier than the chicken legs (again with the skin removed).

- **Eat more fish.** Fish is an excellent alternative to eating red meat. Try to eat fish about three times a week. Fish that contain omega-3 fatty acid has been shown to be helpful in reducing cholesterol and lowering blood pressure. Examples of fish that are high in this fatty acid are tuna, salmon, herring, and mackerel. However, other types of fish are also healthy. Exceptions to this are shrimp and lobster—while they are low in saturated fats, they are high in cholesterol.

- **Use lowfat dairy products.** Use skim milk and 1% milk instead of whole or 2% milk, because they contain the same nutrients without the unnecessary fat and cholesterol. Avoid cream, half-and-half, and even nondairy creamers because they are high in saturated fats. Ice cream contains eggs, whole milk and cream, so eat sherbets and frozen yogurt. Use lowfat or nonfat yogurt instead of sour cream (or try the newer nonfat or lowfat sour creams).

- **Avoid most cheeses.** Most types of cheese contain the same amount of cholesterol as meat but also contain *more* saturated fats and less nutrients than meat. Natural and processed cheeses are the worst; imitation cheeses or those made with skim milk may be lower in fat content but you still need to be careful. Avoid cream cheese—even light cream cheese should be used sparingly. Lowfat cottage cheese is a good choice.

- **Use fats and oils sparingly.** Avoid butter, lard, fatback, shortening, and mayonnaise. Use margarine made from polyunsaturated vegetable oils in a tub rather than in stick form. Use oils such as olive, canola, corn, or vegetable oil when cooking, but use even these sparingly. Avoid products that contain coconut, palm, or peanut oil and peanut butter. Creamy salad dressings should also be avoided.

- **Cut back on snacks and baked goods.** Generally speaking, baked goods contain too much saturated fat and cholesterol. Avoid foods such as doughnuts, cakes, pies, croissants, and cupcakes. You can substitute store-bought baked goods (including ready-to-bake items) with homemade recipes using egg whites or skim milk, and so on. Try eating fruits, popsicles, or raisins as a snack.

Remember that changing your eating habits can be difficult to maintain if you do it all at once. So, start by cutting things out of your diet slowly. Then, gradually increase your intake of the following types of foods—they'll help fill you up as you cut back on meat and other high-fat foods:

- **Foods that are high in fiber.** Increasing your intake of dietary fiber (especially soluble fibers) to 20–25 grams per day has been shown to reduce blood cholesterol and the risk for some forms of cancer. In addition, it may have an effect on blood sugar and blood pressure. Oats, in particular, have been shown to be the most effective—eating two ounces of oats per day along with a lowfat diet can decrease your cholesterol level. Examples of foods with soluble fibers are oatmeal, broccoli, brussels sprouts, grapefruit, apples, and navy beans. Foods with insoluble fibers, such as whole-wheat foods, asparagus, and peas, are good for maintaining regularity.

- **Breads and cereals.** These are low in fat, and high in fiber. When buying bread from a store, make sure that it is made with unsatu-

Table 8.1   Choices in Meat

Meat	Avoid	Choose
Beef	Steaks: ribs, club, porterhouse, T-bone Roasts: rib roast Pot roasts: shoulder, chuck blade, short ribs, brisket, short plate	Steaks: flank, top round, fat-trimmed tenderloin, sirloin Roasts: fat-trimmed tenderloin, top round, eye of round, rump sirloin Pot roasts: rolled flank, fat-trimmed bottom round, chuck arm or shank
Veal	Steaks: rib chops Roasts: shoulder, rib, breast Pot roasts: breast	Steaks: round steak, loin chops or cutlets Roasts: round, rump, sirloin Pot roasts: shoulder, arm, shank
Lamb	Steaks: rib chops Roasts: rib, loin, shoulder Pot roasts: breast, shoulder	Steaks: centerbone leg steaks, fat-trimmed loin chops Roasts: fat-trimmed leg of lamb Pot roasts: shank
Pork and Ham	Steaks: rib chops, spare ribs, bacon Roasts: picnic, shoulder, rib-end roast Pot roasts: shoulder, blade, ribs, hocks, jowl, feet	Steaks: fresh or cured ham slice (pork leg steak), center-cut pork chops or loin cutlets, all fat-trimmed Roasts: fat-trimmed fresh or smoked ham, tenderloin, center-cut loin Pot roasts: fat-trimmed fresh or smoked bottom or rump, arm of picnic, cured ham

rated fats. Do not add a generous amount of butter or margarine to a roll; this will undo the positive effects of eating more bread.

- **Pasta, rice, and dried peas and beans (legumes).** Mix these items with a smaller portion of meat and you can have a filling, nutritious meal. Don't use creamy sauces or butter when eating pasta or rice. Legumes, such as lentils or beans, are very nutritious, low in fat, and high in fiber.

- **Fruits and vegetables.** Fruits and vegetables are an excellent source of vitamins and fiber while also being lowfat. Avoid using butter or rich cheese or cream sauces with your vegetables.

- **Fluids.** Fluids help flush toxins out of your body, carry nutrients to your cells, keep your skin soft and supple, and curb your appetite since you'll feel fuller more quickly. Be careful about drinking too many caffeinated or sugary drinks like soft drinks.

Refer to table 8.2, adapted from dietary guidelines from the National Cholesterol Education Panel (1988), for the fat and cholesterol content for certain meats, poultry, and fish. You can use this table as a quick reference for what to avoid and healthier alternatives.

You can monitor your daily food intake using the Food Diary on page 106. Be sure to make selections from each food group, with special focus on breads, cereals, rice, pasta, fruits, and vegetables.

The following cooking tips will also help you cut down on your total fat and cholesterol:

- **Purchase a cookbook with heart-healthy recipes and alternative choices to ingredients with higher fat content.** There are many books available that outline in great detail the fat content and cholesterol content of each food as well as other nutritional information. These books also provide healthier alternatives and many recipes of new ways of preparing standard dishes that are more heart-friendly. You may learn new combinations of foods that are equally as delicious as your old favorites.

- **Shop smart and check the ingredients of the food products that you buy.** Food producers are required by law to print information on the packaging about the nutritional content of that food and listing other ingredients used to make the product. A standard food label contains information on serving size, a breakdown of calories, total fat, carbohydrate, and protein content per each serving size. It also provides information on the amount of saturated fat per serving and the percent of calories from fat. This is extremely helpful in making a quick assessment of the food you're about to buy and eat. If it looks to be too high in fat content, buy something else instead of bringing it home and increasing your temptation to eat it. The food labels

Table 8.2   Cholesterol and Fat Content in Meat, Poultry, and Fish

Source	Cholesterol Content (mg/3 oz)	Total Fat Content (g/3 oz)
Red Meats (Lean)		
Beef	77	8.7
Lamb	78	8.8
Pork	79	11.1
Veal	128	4.7
Organ Meats		
Liver	270	4.0
Pancreas (sweetbreads)	400	2.8
Kidney	329	2.9
Brains	1746	10.7
Heart	164	4.8
Poultry		
Chicken (without skin)		
Light	72	3.8
Dark	79	8.2
Turkey (without skin)		
Light	59	1.3
Dark	72	6.1
Fish		
Salmon	74	9.3
Tuna, light, canned in water	55	0.7
Shellfish		
Abalone	90	0.8
Clams	57	1.7
Crab Meat		
Alaska King	45	1.3
Blue crab	85	1.5
Lobster	61	0.5
Oysters	93	4.2
Scallops	35	0.8
Shrimp	166	0.9

will also provide you with information on vitamins and minerals present in the food. Ingredient lists will tell you the types of oils, added sugars and salts, and so on. The closer the ingredient is to the beginning of the list, the more of it there is in the product.

- **Broil, bake, poach, roast, or braise your meat and poultry.** Do not fry your meats, as this usually requires adding extra oil. Trim off as much fat as you can before cooking. Remove skin from poultry. When roasting, place the meat on a rack so the fat may drip down into a pan.

- **Steam or sauté vegetables without adding extra oil. Season the vegetables with herbs and spices instead of butter or rich sauces.**

- **Use nonstick cookware.** Use a cooking oil spray to lightly coat the pan as needed.

- **Try flavored vinegars and use lowfat salad dressings on salads.** Use smaller amounts of oil in dressings.

- **When making a soup or stew, let it cool in the refrigerator and spoon off the solidified fat from the top before you reheat and eat.** Fat will float to the top, which makes it easy to remove the excess.

- **Try some of the new lowfat and nonfat products that are available now.** Due to increasing awareness of healthy eating, food producers are presenting alternatives that are equally as flavorful without the added fat.

The Role of Salt and High Blood Pressure

Salt is dangerous to your heart especially if you have high blood pressure. Your body needs a little sodium (salt) in order to keep a certain amount of fluids. But excess salt causes your body to retain excess fluid, which then collects in places in your body including arteries and veins. The more fluid there is in your body, the higher your blood pressure. And as you know, higher blood pressure puts extra strain on your heart. The recommended amount of salt that should be consumed per day is about 2000–3000 mg. Consider the following tips to help reduce your sodium intake:

- **Check the label of foods for the amount of sodium in them.** Other words for salt include monosodium glutamate (MSG), sodium nitrate, sodium chloride, sodium propionate, sea salt, and kelp.

- **Reduce your intake of processed foods.** Packaged foods, frozen dinners, canned soups, and dressings are all high in sodium. Fast food is also high in sodium.

- **Cut down on high-sodium condiments.** Condiments such as pickles, ketchup, mustard, and soy sauce are high in sodium. Try lemon juice, salt substitute, and other spices.

- **Do not salt your food at the table.** It is likely that there is already enough salt in the food.

- **Increase your potassium intake.** Eat more potassium in the form of one extra serving per day of a fresh fruit or vegetable such as a banana, baked potato, or an eight-ounce glass of orange or grapefruit juice.

If you have a serious problem with high blood pressure, then consult with your physician and a dietitian for specific guidelines.

The Role of Being Overweight

One of the risk factors for heart disease is being overweight, especially obesity. Excess weight is not only associated with higher cholesterol levels, but it forces the heart to pump harder to maintain the extra weight as it increases blood pressure and the risk of having diabetes, all of which are risk factors for heart disease. By losing excess weight, it's possible to decrease your cholesterol and triglyceride levels, increase your HDL cholesterol level, and lower your blood pressure. Using the methods for watching your fat intake, plus exercising, is your best way to lose weight. Crash dieting will not only be unhealthy for you, but ineffective in keeping the weight off permanently when your body tries to regain what you have deprived it. A combination of healthy eating and exercise will keep your energy and mood up, which is necessary when dealing with any stress or illness.

Tips for Eating Out

When you're watching what you eat, eating out can be especially difficult. Fast food restaurant chains have been successful in providing quick and easy access to a high-fat, high-sodium meal. The odds are that you live within a one- or two-mile radius of several fast food restaurants. Consider the calories, fat, and sodium in one order of McDonald's Big Mac and small fries: 794 calories, 46 grams of fat, and almost 1000 mg of sodium. Fast food restaurants have recently introduced the concept of supersizing: for slightly more money, you can get a special meal of larger portions with more calories, more fat, and more sodium. And this is only for one meal! Limit how often you eat at fast food restaurants to "almost never." If you must eat there, eat any healthier alternatives they may offer, such as broiled chicken sandwiches without mayonnaise or salads. And if you're absolutely stuck, limit your portions to the small sizes.

Food Diary

For three days, keep track of how many servings you have of each of these food categories. For each category, divide the total servings by three to get your daily average for the period. Compare your eating pattern to the ideal.

	Day One Servings	Day Two Servings	Day Three Servings	Average Servings per day	Ideal Servings per day
Vegetables and Fruits (serving = ½ cup, 1 apple, 1 orange, medium potato)					4
Bread and Cereals (serving = 1 slice bread, ¾ cup cereal)					4
Milk, Cheese, Yogurt (serving = 1 cup milk, 1 medium slice cheese)					2–4
Meat, Poultry, Fish, Eggs, Beans, Nuts (serving = 3 oz. lean meat, two eggs, 1¼ cup cooked beans, 4 Tbsp. peanut butter, ¾ cup nuts)					2
Alcohol (serving = 1 beer, 1 glass of wine or cocktail)					0–1
Fats and Sweets (serving = 1 candy bar, 2 Tbsp. salad dressing, 1 cup ice cream, 1 order french fries)					0
Caffeine (serving = 1 cup coffee or black tea)					0

When eating out at other types of restaurants, you have more opportunity to make healthier choices for yourself. Many restaurants offer heart-healthy options on their menus and mark them as such. You also have the right to ask how something is prepared, what type of sauce is used, and so on. Remember to ask for sauces and dressings to be served on the side, and meat and fish to be grilled, broiled, baked, or poached. Avoid cream or cheese sauces and ask if vegetables are steamed with no butter. Eat half a portion of a richer dish by sharing with your dinner partner. Ethnic restaurants like Chinese, Indian, Thai, Italian, and Mexican often have many meat dishes that have been adapted here to suit American's love of meat and fat. But their more original dishes are actually higher in complex carbohydrates with meat being an addition. Find a favorite ethnic restaurant that offers delicious choices that are lower in fat. Just remember, being educated and aware of what you're eating will help you maintain a healthy diet.

The Benefits of Red Wine and Alcohol

The effects of alcohol, particularly red wine, on heart disease were noted first in countries such as France and Italy where the diet is moderately rich, but where red wine is consumed every day with a meal. It was noted that the expected incidence of heart disease was actually lower. It has been shown that alcohol, in *moderate* amounts, can raise the level of HDL cholesterol. However, too much alcohol clearly carries dangers of its own, including high triglyceride levels, liver damage, increased risk of developing some cancers, birth defects if consumed while pregnant, and psychological and social problems. If you choose to drink alcohol, do so in moderation—no more than one or two servings per day. Recent studies are also examining whether red grape juice provides similar benefits as red wine.

Maintaining Your Commitment to a Healthy Diet

As with anything that requires motivation and a commitment to lifestyle changes, it is essential to believe in the immediate health benefits of reducing your cholesterol and fat intake and in your own ability to make that change. Many people with prior cardiac disease report that they maintain their motivation and commitment to their diets by visualizing the positive benefits in their body. Let's face it, if you view your diet as restrictive, boring, and without any real immediate benefit, you're less likely to remain true to it. The benefits of following a strict, lowfat diet are compelling: in his best-selling book, *Reversing Heart Disease* (1990), Dr. Dean Ornish had the participants

of his program on a strict lowfat, low cholesterol diet in combination
with moderate exercise and stress management. The participants already had significant narrowing or blockage of their arteries. Pre-
and posttesting done with magnetic resonance imaging (MRI) scans
showed an actual *reversal of the narrowing of their arteries.* If this type
of strict eating produced such dramatic results, then imagine the impact on your heart health you could gain by monitoring what you
eat—even if not as stringently as Dr. Ornish's program.

Much of the information about diet and exercise presented in
this chapter may not be totally new for you. Heard it, done it, been
there, but can't seem to stick with it. Does this sound familiar? You
are not alone. If you've already suffered a heart attack, are a family
member of someone who has cardiac disease, or are simply trying
to keep your heart healthy, then you know that making these two
basic lifestyle changes is not easy. Many of the cardiac patients and
their families that we work with describe a turning point in their
compliance or follow-through with the diet and exercise. Initially,
many people hear the information but need to test the waters. They
experiment and ask themselves questions: "How restrictive do I have
to be with what I eat and still stay healthy?" "Will the exercise really
make a difference for my heart?" Each of these questions reflects a
need for most people to see and believe that immediate health benefits
are occurring. If your body were transparent, it would make believing
much easier. However, until scientists can make this a reality, you
can only rely on your imagery skills and positive messages. When
you effectively use these skills, you may find that you've reached
this turning point where your commitment to your diet and exercise
is renewed.

Imagery exercises, which can help you keep focused on the benefits to your body, can help you sustain your motivation. Also, how
you view your diet and the role that you believe foods play in your
well-being are important factors in your commitment to changing
your eating patterns. The following visualization exercises are designed to help you imagine what is happening inside your body when
you are eating certain foods that are high in saturated fat and cholesterol. These imagery exercises can be used to encourage and support your efforts to eat healthy and exercise regularly.

Let's first examine the use of imagery skills: A powerful motivator for change is the belief that the energy you're expending is going
to be worthwhile. For medical patients, worthwhile usually refers to
seeing or experiencing immediate improvements to their health. Imagining changes to your body with your diet and exercise is one way
of seeing these benefits to your health. Try using the illustration in
figure 8.2 to visualize the reduction of your LDL cholesterol with
each bite of lowfat food that you eat. Imagine cholesterol as packages
leaving your liver. The package of LDL cholesterol and triglycerides

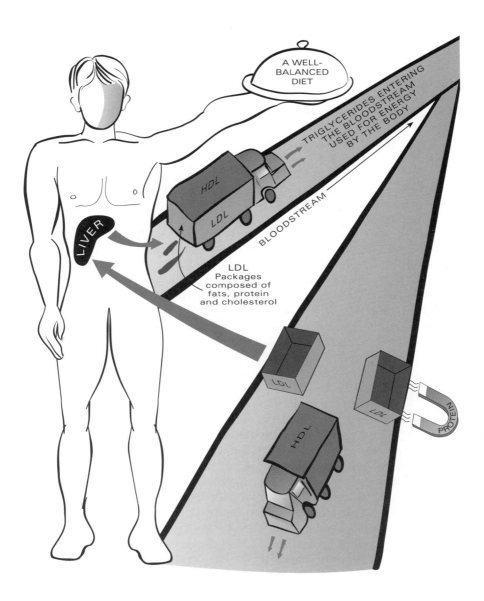

Figure 8.2   A Healthy Diet

enters the bloodstream. As you eat a healthy diet, just the right amount of packages are released by the liver. They readily and comfortably flow through the river of blood in your arteries. As the packages are circulating, some will be drawn to protein molecules and carried off in your body to do healthy work. Your healthy cholesterol then comes along like an athletic, strong rescuer carrying the leftover cholesterol back to the liver before it can stick to the lining of the arteries. As you continue to eat healthy, you prevent bad cholesterol from getting backed up and blocking your arteries.

Conversely, you may need to imagine that your artery is clogged up as if it were clamped shut by the large amount of LDL cholesterol in your blood with each bite of fatty food that you eat. Use the illustration in figure 8.3 to imagine what happens when you eat fatty foods. With each bite of high-fat food that you eat, too many packages of cholesterol will be flowing through your blood. The HDL will not be able to pick up all of the excess cholesterol, and your blood will become crowded. The excess cholesterol then begins to stick to the walls of your arteries. Imagine your arteries slowly narrowing, making it difficult for your blood to flow smoothly.

The same imagery can be applied when exercising. Try imagining as you walk or swim that your HDL cholesterol level is increasing and is therefore better able to carry the LDL cholesterol out of the blood before it can clog your arteries. Think of figure 8.3; it showed how LDL can accumulate in your bloodstream when you consume foods that are high in saturated fat. The blood becomes "crowded," and this prevents the easy flow of blood through the arteries. Your diet is the primary source of this crowding of LDL because the more fat you eat the more LDLs are made by the liver.

On a final note, getting support from those around you will be immensely helpful in making this lifestyle change. Changing to a healthy diet will benefit everyone in your family, and there will be less temptation for you if they, too, agree to some of these changes. If you have growing children in the house whose nutritional needs may differ, compromise by having healthy alternatives for yourself. If some members of your family refuse to change their diets completely, and you feel constantly tempted by the types of "wrong" foods that are making their way to your house, ask them if they would be willing to eat these foods away from your presence. You cannot control what others choose to do, but you do have control over the choices that you make.

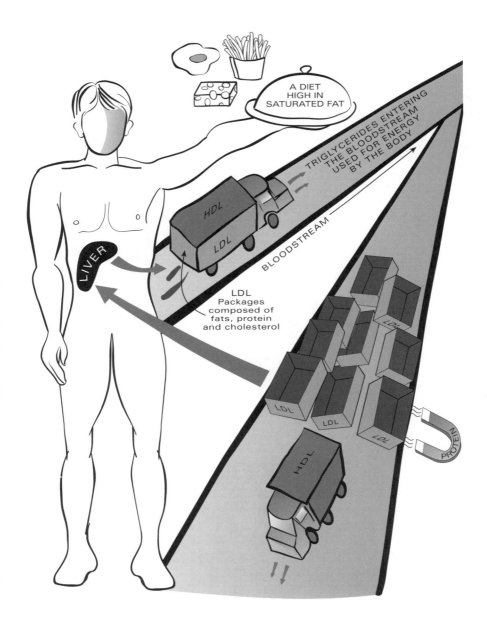

Figure 8.3   A Diet High in Saturated Fats

9

Exercising

Exercise is one of the best activities that can be added to your life. For cardiac patients, exercise is even more important because of the benefits to cardiovascular health. In 1993, the American Heart Association specifically included having a sedentary lifestyle as a major risk factor for coronary heart disease. Exercise can help your heart in the following ways:

- Increase your heart's ability to pump oxygen-rich blood to parts of your body

- Reduce high blood pressure

- Increase your body's level of HDL cholesterol, the "good" cholesterol

- Decrease your body's level of LDL cholesterol, the "bad" cholesterol, by keeping your overall weight and body fat down

Exercise is also one of the best things you can do for your body in times of stress. When you read chapter 15, you'll see that how you manage stress is very important in maintaining good heart health. The extra tension in the fight-or-flight response that was triggered in our ancestors was essential to their survival. But that extra tension was released by some physical response like running or fighting for survival. In current times, the same stress response is triggered by events every day, but we usually do not have a chance to discharge this physical tension at the moment, at least not in ways that are socially appropriate. For instance, having an important meeting at work can trigger a stress response, but you may end up keeping the physical tension bottled up inside. When the pressure begins to build from several different stressors, your body will start to wear out.

Exercise can provide the opportunity to release this tension. This is particularly important for people who suffer from cardiac disease because the body's response to stress, as you recall, involves the heart having to work harder in order to supply more oxygen to the body.

The basic mechanism of exercise, which improves your heart function, is that when your body exerts itself by using muscles, those muscles demand more oxygen. Your heart has to pump harder to keep up with the oxygen requirements. With continued regular activity, your muscles become more efficient at getting the oxygen they need from the blood and subsequently, your heart does not have to work as hard and your heart rate becomes reduced. The average heart beats seventy times per minute at rest. A heart that has been conditioned through exercise can supply the body with the same amount of oxygen with fewer heartbeats.

There are numerous other physical and psychological benefits of exercise. Research continues to show that regular exercise, even in moderate amounts, can improve your overall health. As with any lifestyle change that was not previously part of your routine, maintaining your motivation to keep up an exercise program can be difficult. Reminding yourself of the some of the following benefits may be helpful. Exercise

- Can help fight weight gain
- Improves muscle strength, flexibility, and endurance
- Reduces muscle aches and tension
- Reduces potential for back problems
- Increases energy level, and reduces fatigue
- Improves digestion and bowel functioning
- Increases production of endorphins, your body's natural substance that improves your mood, promotes a feeling of well-being, and combats pain
- Improves sleeping habits
- Helps in managing stress more effectively
- Improves resistance to illness
- Improves self-esteem
- Decreases feelings of depression or anxiety

Starting an Exercise Program

If you've been diagnosed with heart disease, already suffered a heart attack, or have chest pain, it is of the utmost importance that you *consult with your physician prior to beginning any type of exercise program.*

This is important because without proper exercise training first, doing activities that significantly raise your heart rate can be dangerous to a heart that is damaged. If you have coronary arteries that are narrowed due to atherosclerosis, your heart is already working hard to get the oxygen that it needs. Taxing it even further can lead to chest pain or worse. Your physician can recommend an exercise program that is right for you.

If you've had a heart attack or frequent chest pain, the idea of exercising can be anxiety-provoking. It is a legitimate concern to have, since vigorous exercise does stress the heart. You may have experienced chest pain during your stress EKG test, or you may have suffered your heart attack while you were exerting yourself in some way. It is not uncommon for heart attacks to occur after a person has been doing some strenuous activity. Therefore, consciously forcing yourself to raise your heart rate through exercise with the threat of experiencing chest discomfort or worse is daunting.

This anxiety can be alleviated by first having a thorough evaluation done by your physician with strict recommendations and guidelines for an exercise regimen. Further, a referral to a cardiac rehabilitation program can be extremely beneficial and is strongly advised. Cardiac rehabilitation programs have an exercise component built in, with trained exercise physiologists (experts in exercise and its interactions with the body). These professionals will monitor you closely and help you condition your heart at a slow, gradual, and safe pace. The constant supervision means they will be alert to any discomfort that may be potentially dangerous to your heart. They can design a specific exercise program that is safe for you. The major goal of the exercise program in cardiac rehabilitation is to maintain your heart rate within an acceptable range and increase your endurance without causing any symptoms of heart problems. The signs or symptoms that are monitored do not only include angina (chest pain) or your EKG results, but general fatigue as well. The exercise physiologist can provide encouragement when your motivation is waning and reassurance if you feel particularly anxious.

Before you begin exercising in a cardiac rehabilitation or prevention program, you will undergo an exercise stress test, or stress EKG, to determine your individual exercise intensity and the level at which you begin to show changes on your EKG patterns (that is, the level of exercise at which your heart begins to show strain). Exercise intensity is measured by your maximum heart rate during exercise. During a stress EKG, the maximum heart rate is the number of heartbeats per minute at your highest comfortable pace. Your maximum heart rate can also be calculated by subtracting your age from 220. For example, if you are 45 years old, your estimated maximum heart rate is $220 - 45 = 175$ beats per minute. If you exercised close to this level, you would become exhausted quickly and become prone to injury. The more appropriate target range is 60 to 80 percent of your maximum heart rate; however, you may find that starting at an exercise intensity level that gets your heart pumping at 45 percent of its maximum heart rate is more comfortable and safer. Remember, if you've already been diagnosed with cardiac disease, please proceed with caution under your doctor's guidance.

Experts recommend that you exercise to the point of raising your heart rate into a target range for about twenty minutes, with another five minutes on either end for warming up and cooling down. The exercise should be aerobic, which means moving your limbs actively against low resistance (for example, swimming or bicycling), rather than anaerobic exercise, which is moving against high resistance (for example, weightlifting). Aerobic exercise increases your body's intake of oxygen and helps your body become more efficient in its use of oxygen. If you're not used to this type of exercise and are just getting started, exercise for as many minutes as you can. When you feel that you can exercise for five to ten minutes comfortably, then slowly add more time each week until you can sustain at least thirty minutes of aerobic exercise. You can measure your heart rate per minute by checking your pulse for ten seconds and multiplying that number by six. To check your pulse, place the tips of the first two fingers lightly on the inside of your wrist right below the base of your thumb, or on the left or right carotid arteries in your neck (located right under your jaw on either side of your neck). It's important to check your heart rate during exercise, so take your pulse when you are actively exercising or immediately after stopping. If you're in a cardiac rehabilitation program, you may be asked to wear a monitor. Don't be concerned if your heart rate is not in the target range yet. With time and continued exercising, it will get there. If you're inconsistent with your exercising, it will take longer to get in shape and you may feel that exercise is more tiring.

Refer to table 9.1 for heart rate target zones for people aged twenty to eighty-five years.

The Importance of Stretching, Warming Up, and Cooling Down

It is important to prepare your body gradually rather than launching right into a faster pace of exercise. This will help reduce the chance of injuries to your muscles. Take about five minutes to warm up your body and do stretching exercises. Begin slowly and in a steady manner. Here are four ways of stretching:

- **Touch your toes.** Stand with your knees slightly bent and feet apart. Bend from the waist and try to touch your fingers to the floor or to your ankles. Count to ten while holding this position.

Repeat the exercise once or twice. Make sure you do not bounce. If you have low back problems, try this exercise with your legs crossed.

- **Push against a wall.** Stand one or two feet away from a wall. Lean forward and while keeping your heels flat, push your palms against the wall. Count to ten, rest, and repeat one or two times.

- **Stretch your shoulders and arms.** Reach back with one arm like you are scratching your shoulder blade. Place the other hand on your elbow to extend the stretch. Alternate your arms and repeat one or two times.

- **Loosen your neck muscles.** Slowly rotate your head from side to front to side. Drop your head to your chest and then slowly raise your head back to look up at the ceiling, being careful not to drop it too far back. Repeat this several times.

After you've completed your exercising, spend a few minutes cooling down by gradually decreasing your pace. If you're swimming, change your pace to a slower one. If you're jogging, cool down by walking for a few minutes. This cooling down will help prevent dizziness and muscle cramping. You may repeat any stretching exercises if you choose.

Table 9.1   Heart Rate Target Zones

Age	Target Zone (beats/minute)		Maximum Heart Rate (100%)
	45–60%	60–80%	
20	90–120	120–160	200
25	88–117	117–156	195
30	85–114	114–152	190
35	83–111	111–148	185
40	80–108	108–144	180
45	77–105	105–140	175
50	74–102	102–136	170
55	71–99	99–132	165
60	69–96	96–128	160
65	66–93	93–124	155
70	63–90	90–120	150
75	60–87	87–116	145
80	57–84	84–112	140
85	54–81	81–108	135

Types of Exercise

There are many ways you can get exercise other than running, jogging, or aerobics at the local health club. If you've received an okay from your doctor and you've gradually increased your exercise tolerance safely, then there are many activities you can do that will exercise your body and keep you interested. Choose some activities from the following list that you used to do or that you might like to do:

_____	Swimming	_____	Dancing
_____	Bowling	_____	Tennis
_____	Baseball	_____	Hiking
_____	Bicycling	_____	Calisthenics
_____	Stationary cycling	_____	Golf
_____	Fast walking	_____	Volleyball
_____	Ice skating	_____	Yoga

Many of the activities you do around the house and everyday errands also give your body exercise. How many of the following did you used to do regularly? Ask your doctor whether these are safe activities for you now:

_____	Washing car	_____	Raking leaves
_____	Gardening	_____	Grocery shopping
_____	Vacuuming	_____	Mowing lawn
_____	Climbing stairs	_____	Walking from parking space to building

The Benefits of Walking

If your doctor has restricted you from vigorous exercise and activities due to the severity of your heart condition, it will nonetheless be important to get some form of exercise in a safe manner. Once again, cardiac rehabilitation programs can be of assistance to you because the staff there will monitor you closely while increasing your exercise tolerance. One of the best ways to exercise safely is walking. Walking is useful for those who are just getting started with exercise and for those who are in poor cardiovascular health. Studies show that moderate exercise, like walking thirty minutes per day or for one hour three times per week, is enough to get your heart in shape and keep you healthy. In his Opening Your Heart program, which showed some reversal of heart disease, Dean Ornish (1990) recommended that participants walk as the primary form of exercise. The other form of exercise he recommended was yoga, both as an exercise to stretch the body and calm the mind. You can take a class at your local community center, buy books, or purchase videos on yoga techniques. And everyone can make the time to walk. Consider the following tips:

- Park a little farther away than usual and walk to your destination.
- Try to walk every place you go.
- Ask a family member or friend to join you for a long walk in the morning or before dinner.
- Go to your local indoor mall in the mornings and join others in a walking program.
- Alternate the places where you walk—sometimes around your neighborhood, sometimes in a park.
- Regularly take your dog, if you have one, for a brisk walk.

A Final Word about Exercise

Exercising is one of the best things you can do for your heart. The increased endurance of your heart will help protect it from suffering another heart attack. However, if you've been diagnosed with heart disease, it's important that you first get a thorough workup from your doctor that includes guidelines for exercising. Keep in mind that you should exercise carefully in excessively warm or cold weather—either extreme makes your heart work harder. You must also use caution and monitor yourself for the following symptoms:

- Excessive fatigue
- Dizziness
- Rapid or irregular heartbeats
- Chest pain that does not go away after resting or after taking nitroglycerin
- Other types of pain or discomfort, like back or arm pain, "indigestion"
- Increased shortness of breath that does not go away
- Muscle or tendon injury

10

Quitting Smoking

In a book that examines emotions, thoughts, and behaviors and their impact on your cardiac health, it is essential to include a chapter on smoking. Most smokers think of smoking as causing damage only to their lungs, if anywhere. However, your heart can be adversely affected by your smoking. Smoking is a major risk factor for cardiovascular disease. There are three primary categories of cardiovascular disease, including coronary heart disease, hypertension, and stroke. Cigarette smoking is a major risk factor for each of these categories.

Coronary heart disease is the leading cause of death in the United States. Smokers have a two to four times greater incidence of developing coronary heart disease and a 70 percent greater chance of dying from heart disease when compared to nonsmokers. Smoking requires the heart to work harder to compensate for the decrease in oxygen caused by carbon monoxide that you inhale with each cigarette. Smoking can also lead to the formation of *plaques*, hard deposits of fatty tissues inside the artery. This makes it difficult for blood to flow easily through the artery.

In addition, emotional states such as depression and anxiety appear to have a large impact on why you smoke and whether or not you feel you can quit smoking. In the sections that follow, we will help you learn more about your smoking, and as a result you will become a more educated consumer of your cigarettes. We will also help you prepare yourself for quitting. By actually keeping a record of your smoking, you will be able to better identify *when* you smoke and *why* you smoke. For example, is driving a car or feeling bored a particular trigger for you to smoke? By identifying your risk factors, you'll learn to substitute smoking with healthy alternative strategies such as stress reduction techniques, imagery, meditation, anger control, and so on, which are detailed in later sections of the book.

Cigarette smoking has probably been a part of your life for quite some time, but do you really know much about it? Sometimes notions and beliefs about something, including smoking, are repeated so often that you come to believe they are facts. Often these so-called facts or myths can be misleading and can contribute to uninformed choices or high-risk behaviors. How much do you really know about cigarette smoking?

Did you know that there are more than four thousand substances in your cigarettes? Most smokers are shocked to discover how many substances they are inhaling and equally stunned at what these substances are. Table 10.1 shows just a few of them. This is in keeping with the goal of making you a more educated consumer of your cigarettes.

Table 10.1   What's in a Cigarette

Substance	Description	Effect on the Body
Tar	Black sticky substance	Adheres to the lungs, making it difficult to breathe
Arsenic	Poisonous gas	
Ammonia	Powerful substance found in cleaning agents	Irritant to throat and nasal passages
Carbon Monoxide	Gas that is emitted from car exhaust pipe	Poisons healthy red blood cells, limiting the amount of oxygen to organs
Hydrogen Cyanide	Substance used in gas chamber to kill	
Formaldehyde	Substance used to embalm dead bodies	Toxic to cilia in the lungs, limiting their ability to clear poisons from the lungs
Asbestos	Fiberlike substance used for insulating, now banned	Adheres to the lungs
PO210	Radioactive substance found in fertilizers used on tobacco	Generally toxic to all organs in the body
Cyanide	Deadly poison	
Lead	Substance that has been banned from paint and plumbing	Associated with neurological damage

| DDT | Deadly pesticide | Poisonous |
| Acetaldehyde | First-degree metabolite of Ethanol | Poisonous to the cells of the heart |

A habit is something that you do automatically without even consciously thinking. The goal here is to get you to consciously think about each cigarette you smoke. Imagine your body as transparent. With each drag off your cigarette, try to envision and track all four thousand substances as they enter your body. Now, look at figure 10.1 to see what actually happens in your body while smoking. Figure 10.2 shows what happens specifically to your heart when you smoke. Although this can be frightening and overwhelming, the purpose is to make you aware of smoking's effects on your body.

Remember from chapter 7 that if you believe you are susceptible to an illness and you believe that your behavior is having immediate effects on your health, you are more likely to be motivated to change. It is often difficult to believe the negative health messages you hear, particularly if you are in good health. However, you may not necessarily be healthy simply because you are not currently experiencing any symptoms.

How Your Smoking Habit Began

It's important to understand how your smoking has developed into a habit and how you continue to maintain this habit. Only then can you break away from being a helpless victim of this habit. Changing a habit requires awareness and active participation on your part. This chapter will help you get your smoking more under your control.

How does smoking *become* a habit in the first place? Basically, by being associated or linked with all of your everyday activities, emotions, and situations. But it was not *always* linked with everything that you did. Take a closer look at how your smoking habit began.

Do you remember your first cigarette? In the space provided below, please describe what it was like to smoke your first cigarette: How old were you? Who were you with? Remember the physical sensations—was it pleasant or did you cough? Did your throat burn?

_____

_____

_____

_____

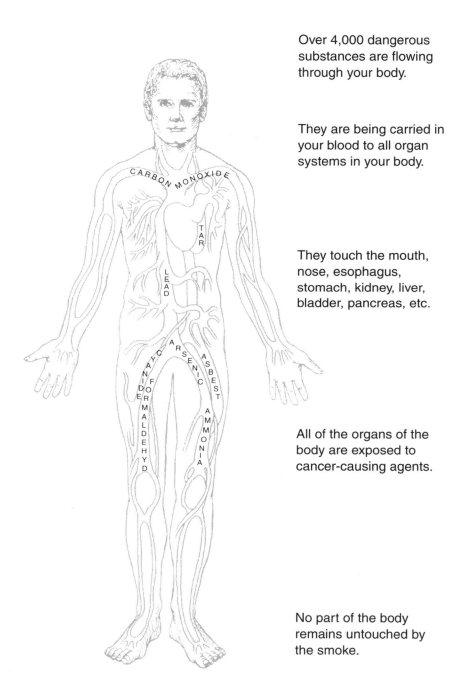

Over 4,000 dangerous substances are flowing through your body.

They are being carried in your blood to all organ systems in your body.

They touch the mouth, nose, esophagus, stomach, kidney, liver, bladder, pancreas, etc.

All of the organs of the body are exposed to cancer-causing agents.

No part of the body remains untouched by the smoke.

Figure 10.1   What Happens When You Smoke?

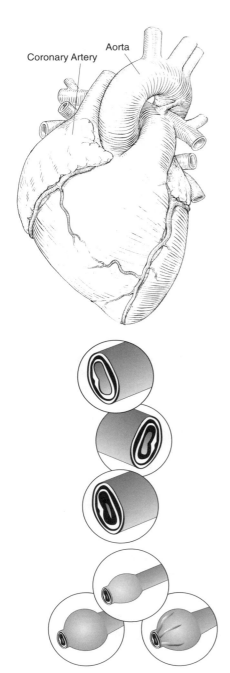

Immediately after you inhale your cigarette, your blood pressure increases by 10 to 20 points.

Blood vessels in the brain can become clogged and stop blood flow, which can result in a stroke.

The heart can become discolored from the black tar.

This increase in your heart rate and blood pressure increases your body's need for oxygen and therefore your heart must work much harder.

Although your body needs more oxygen, the carbon monoxide from your cigarette decreases the amount of oxygen that can get into your body. This can lead to chest pain or heart attack.

The cigarette smoke can contribute to the formation of plaques and other fatty substances on the inside lining of the arteries in your heart.

This leads to a narrowing or closing off of blood flow to the heart. This can lead to a heart attack.

When your blood pressure increases, the strain on your arteries is great.

Not only is blood trying to pass through a narrow opening, but it is doing so under great pressure.

This can result in the artery rupturing and bleeding.

Figure 10.2 Smoking and Your Cardiovascular System (Your Heart)

Did one or both of your parents smoke? Other family members? Friends?

_____

_____

_____

Why and when did you smoke again? How do you remember feeling
—cool? More grown-up? Describe how you see yourself now as a
smoker—for example, more confident? Self-assured?

_____

_____

_____

_____

Typically, smokers report that they smoked their first cigarette
during late childhood or during their teenage years. They either imi-
tated a family member (years of watching Dad or Mom smoke) or
a friend encouraged them to try one. But many smokers also report
that smoking their first cigarette was not a pleasant experience! You,
too, may have coughed a lot, your eyes and throat burned. You may
not have even known how to inhale! It was certainly not the same
"pleasant" feeling you may experience now.

You may have found yourself experimenting once or twice per
week or month in spite of the first unpleasant experience because
your friends smoked or it made you feel older. You may have seen
advertisements that showed smokers who were young, beautiful, or
handsome and appeared to have the world at their fingertips. Seeing
your favorite actor or actress smoking also would have had a strong
impact on your decision to see what cigarettes were all about even
though smoking that first one was unpleasant. Soon you may have
been smoking every time you were out with your friends. So cigarettes became linked or associated in your mind with having a good
time and relaxing (since most probably you were having fun with
your friends). Therefore, having a good time or relaxing became a
cue to smoke.

Soon you probably started to smoke at other times—in different
situations or when you were feeling tense or bored. Smoking then
became linked to a wider variety of situations, emotions, and people
in your life. These links or associations became strengthened through
thousands of repetitions (as your smoking increased to one or two
packs per day multiplied by several years). Situations, emotions, and
people became cues or triggers to smoke a cigarette. For example,

how often do you think of a cup of coffee with a cigarette? A cigarette when you start the car? A cigarette after you finish a meal and lean back in your chair? Or how about a cigarette after a hard day's work or after an argument? By now, these activities probably seem to naturally "fit" together like salt and pepper, peanut butter and jelly. Smoking fits with these activities because you've paired them together hundreds, maybe thousands, of times. Therefore, drinking a cup of coffee, getting in the car, and leaning back in your chair after a meal serve as cues to get a cigarette. Reaching for a cigarette also becomes natural when you feel anxious, angry, or socially awkward.

The following exercises will help you further understand how these cues maintain your smoking habit and how they have become part of your daily life without you being consciously aware of them.

Read the following scenarios and mark which ones apply to you:

_____ You've just finished your favorite dinner; you push your plate away and reach for a cigarette.

_____ While you're waiting in the cashier's line at your local drugstore, you spot the cigarette stand with your favorite brand. You decide to buy a carton.

_____ You are under a lot of pressure at work to finish a project. You know the pressure will continue for a while. A cigarette might ease the pressure so that you may work better.

_____ You're waiting at a restaurant for a friend who is half an hour late. You've already ordered a drink. You think a cigarette would help pass the time.

_____ You've just picked up your car from the mechanic and the bill is much higher than you expected it to be. As you drive home, you find that the very problem you took the car in for is still not fixed, and it stalls at a light. You feel angry and frustrated: you need a cigarette.

_____ You've had a stressful, hectic day at work—everybody needed something from you, and it seemed as though you would never get caught up with your work. Finally, you get home but you are still tense from work. A cigarette would help relax you.

_____ You're at a party with friends. Others are smoking and drinking. You have a glass of wine in your hand and you're laughing and having fun. You always have a cigarette with a drink.

_____ You're on your way to a job interview, and a traffic jam on the highway may make you late. You start to feel anxious and a cigarette would calm your nerves.

_____ You're home alone with nothing to really do; nothing seems interesting—so you reach for cigarette.

_____ You're sitting on your deck with some friends having a barbecue on a warm summer evening. You are relaxed and having a good time. One of your friends lights a cigarette, which looks so refreshing to you.

(Adapted from Shiffman et al., 1983, Smoking Situational Competency Test)

Most smokers check almost all of the above scenarios or situations. You, too, probably smoke on most of these occasions. As we stated before, feeling nervous, angry, or frustrated becomes a trigger to smoke in order to feel better. The preceding situations can be grouped into some common categories that serve as cues for most smokers to get a cigarette. These include

- Eating and/or food substitution: Smoking while drinking coffee or after meals; also, smoking to keep from eating too much and gaining weight

- Negative feelings: Smoking when feeling angry, tense, worried or frustrated; smoking seems to make bad feelings better

- Positive feelings: Some smokers like to smoke when feeling good so that they will feel even better

- Boredom: Smoking is something to do, and the stimulating effects of nicotine help alleviate boredom

- Social: Smoking helps combat any awkwardness in social situations by giving hands something to do; improves self-image (increases confidence because smoker believes he looks more self-assured); also, seeing other smokers serves as cue to smoke

- Alcohol: Commonly associated with smoking

While there may be other situations not described here in which you smoke, the exercise should help you understand that almost everything you do, feel, or experience every day has become associated with smoking—so much so that smoking is now an automatic habit. So, if you've tried to quit in the past and were successful for only a short period of time, it's not necessarily because your body needed the nicotine and you couldn't help yourself. Yes, it is true that you were physically addicted to nicotine. Each time you inhaled, you received a "hit" of nicotine, which means that nicotine was absorbed into your bloodstream. As you continued to smoke over time, your body demanded more of the nicotine. This is how the physical addiction strengthens the psychological addiction.

However, nicotine will leave your body after only a few days. Your craving for cigarettes is not so much physical as it is psychological—your everyday life contains several cues and triggers reminding you to smoke. In your past attempts to quit, you may not have broken these automatic links. You will have more success in staying off cigarettes if you can first recognize the psychological aspects of your habit and then begin to break those links.

This next exercise is an important one in helping you identify your own smoking patterns. Approaching quitting in a systematic manner will help make the whole process more manageable. Please look at the chart on the following page. This is what is referred to by behavioral therapists as a self-monitoring form. The concept of self-monitoring simply involves keeping a daily record of your smoking habit. It serves several purposes: It will give you a more objective picture of exactly how much you smoke. It will provide information about when you tend to smoke more; examining the situations in which you smoke helps identify your feelings at the time (for example, frustrated, bored). Monitoring your own smoking will help you identify where your trouble spots are so that you can anticipate even before quitting when you're likely to really "need a cigarette" and substitute an alternate coping strategy. Also, by monitoring your smoking, you make an unconscious act a more conscious one and by doing so will eliminate those automatic and least important cigarettes from your routine.

Make several copies of the following chart. Fold one copy and wrap it around your cigarettes. When you have the urge to smoke, take out the chart and fill it in before you light the cigarette.

Filling In the Chart

In the far left corner, you'll see a column entitled "Cigarette #." Fill in which number cigarette you are smoking. For each cigarette you smoke, check how you are feeling and the situation you are in. If the feelings listed do not accurately describe your own feelings at the time, feel free to fill in your own description. For example, the next cigarette you smoke will be cigarette number 1. If you are at work, check the column marked "Work"; if you are just finishing a meal, then check the column marked "Eating" or "Drinking Alcohol." Also, include with cigarette number 1 how you are feeling. If you find yourself experiencing symptoms of anxiety, check the column marked "Nervous." If you find yourself feeling bored, then check the column marked "Bored." If none of these feelings or situations apply to you, add your own description. As you can see, you may have several check marks in the row marked cigarette number 1. Now that you've identified what you're doing and what feeling you're experiencing, it's time to rate how important this cigarette is to you.

In the far right column of the chart, you'll see a column marked "How Important Is This Cigarette?" This is your "need rating," in which 1 represents that this cigarette is most important to you, and 4 indicates that this cigarette is being smoked out of habit and is not that important. If you rated the cigarette 1 or 2, indicating that you

Daily Smoking Record

Cig. #	Situation/Place					Activity					Feeling							How Important Is This Cigarette? Very Important 1 Smoke the Cigarette	2	Not Very Important 3	4 Do Not Smoke the Cigarette
	Work	Home	Car	Bar	Other (Where?)	Eating	Watching TV	Drinking Alcohol	Drinking Coffee	Other (What?)	Angry	Bored	Depressed	Sad	Nervous	Relaxed	Other (How?)				

strongly feel the need to smoke the cigarette, go ahead and smoke it. If you rated the cigarette a number 3 or 4, indicating that you probably could do without this cigarette, if even for a while, hold off on smoking it. Put some time between this cigarette and your next one.

Do this for each cigarette that you smoke now until your quit date. And remember, if you have time to smoke your cigarette, you have time to fill in the chart. No excuses.

After one or two weeks of filling in the charts, you'll see your smoking pattern emerge. For example, you may tend to smoke more when you're at work or more when you feel depressed. These times and feeling states become your "high risk" areas, which will need to be addressed before quitting. You'll also notice that merely by keeping track of your cigarettes and eliminating the least important ones (the 3s and 4s), you'll automatically cut down on your smoking. You'll need to refer back to these charts when you are practicing alternative coping strategies such as relaxation or distraction.

Preparing to Quit

Quitting smoking requires preparation. Begin by first choosing your quit date; pick a date within the next two weeks. Then mark this date on a visible calendar. This will serve as a reminder to you that the act of quitting smoking is not something you are doing on a whim but rather something that you are planning to accomplish.

As you approach the date marked on your calendar, you must prepare yourself for the actual quitting process. Since smoking has been part of your whole existence including your physical self, your emotional self, and part of your general surroundings, each of these areas needs preparation for the quitting process.

Prepare Your Surroundings

Cigarette smoking has been part of your life and as such has probably left its mark all around you. In your efforts to quit smoking it is important for you to remove the evidence and reminders of your smoking habit. This will serve to decrease temptation from these reminders as well as strengthen your commitment to the quitting process.

- **Two weeks prior to quit date, limit your smoking to one room in your home.** This room should be the LEAST comfortable place. Move all of your smoking paraphernalia to that room. Limiting where you smoke will help you to cut down on the quantity of cigarettes you are smoking by making the process more inconvenient.

- **Clean out your car.** Remove all evidence that you smoked in your car. Vacuum the carpet, remove the ashtray and lighter, and discard any remaining cigarettes. After your car is clean, make this a nonsmoking area for yourself and other guests who ride in your car. By preparing your car, you will begin to break any associations that you may have between driving your car and smoking a cigarette. Also, as a nonsmoking area your car will become a safe haven for you when you are tempted to smoke.

- **Clean and deodorize your home.** Since you have now limited your smoking to only one room in your home, you can begin to clean and prepare the remaining rooms for your actual quit date. Get your carpets and drapery cleaned. Remove the odor of cigarettes from your furniture and clothing.

Prepare Your Physical Self

Since nicotine is a physically addicting chemical, your body may experience some withdrawal symptoms after you quit smoking. These physical symptoms may include

- Restlessness
- Irritability
- Difficulty concentrating
- Sleep disturbances
- Increased appetite
- Headache
- Constipation
- Dry mouth or sore throat
- Fatigue
- Coughing
- Nicotine craving

It's important to understand that these symptoms are short-lived, lasting anywhere from one to two weeks. Almost all of the nicotine will be out of your system in two to three days. The amount and type of symptoms that smokers experience is very individual. Some smokers experience *no* physical symptoms, while others report several symptoms. Understanding that these symptoms are temporary and are the body's way of *healing itself* can help turn these negative symptoms into a positive reminder that you are on the path of improving your health. It may be helpful to tell yourself that it's like you are getting the flu or a cold. You know that you may feel bad for a while but with the passage of time, each day you'll be closer to feeling better. View these symptoms as "necessary discomforts" in the healing process. To make the process a little more comfortable, it's important to get yourself physically prepared for these changes.

- **Visit your dentist.** Get your teeth cleaned. This will remind you that you are about to begin life as a nonsmoker. With the tar and nicotine removed from your teeth, you are literally starting fresh.

- **Monitor your alcohol consumption prior to and immediately after quitting.** When you drink alcohol, your inhibitions are decreased and you are therefore more likely to relapse into smoking. For many smokers, alcohol is associated with smoking. So when you have a drink, you may automatically begin thinking about a cigarette, which puts you more at risk for relapsing back into smoking. It may be necessary for you to avoid alcohol during the first couple months after quitting, until you are beyond the most difficult phase, and then slowly reintroduce alcohol consumption back into your life.

- **Reduce your caffeine consumption prior to quitting.** Nicotine acts on the body by changing your metabolism. If you are used to consuming a fair amount of caffeine as a smoker, your body may not be able to tolerate the same amount after you quit smoking. If this is the case, you may experience a jittery/nervous sensation that may not be related to tobacco withdrawal but rather caffeine intoxication. Several weeks before your quit date, begin to reduce your caffeine consumption. Remember, caffeine is not just found in coffee but also in chocolate, soda pop, and so on.

- **Get plenty of rest.** During your first smoke-free week, it's important to get plenty of rest. You probably have been bombarding your body with the nicotine for many years. Once you stop smoking, your body needs time to readjust without the drug, which can be difficult and exhausting for the first couple of weeks. Plenty of rest will help you move through this process with greater ease. Think about this phase as a time for recovery.

- **Drink plenty of fluids.** The readjustment process requires good nutrition and plenty of fluids. Try to drink fruit juices, which tend to cut down on the craving for nicotine.

- **Use healthy oral substitutes.** During the initial few weeks after quitting, it's important to have healthy foods prepared for snacking. For example, keep celery, carrots, raisins, apples, pickles, sunflower seeds, and so on readily available for snacking. These snacks will help you when a craving strikes and you need something oral to satisfy you. However, make sure that the snacks you are choosing are low in calorie and high in bulk. This will help with the craving but minimize the weight gain.

- **Chew sugarless gum and hard candy.** During the first few weeks after you quit smoking your throat may feel dry or you may have a "tickle" cough. Sucking on ice chips, hard candy, or chewing gum can help. Also, you can use the candy or gum as a substitute when you have a craving.

Prepare Your Emotional Self

One of the biggest challenges to quitting smoking is preparing yourself emotionally. Many smokers often feel a sense of loss when thinking about quitting smoking. You may find yourself equating quitting smoking with losing a friend or, at the very least, losing your coping strategy. Either way you describe it, there is a sense of loss, security, and control when you quit smoking. To overcome these feelings, you need to prepare yourself emotionally for the process of quitting smoking and life after cigarettes.

- **Repeat to yourself your reasons for *needing* to quit smoking.** Your reasons for needing to quit smoking are what will provide you with the strength and willpower to get through the quitting process. Review these reasons. Reinforce them to yourself several times a day.

- **Plan activities for your first smoke-free week.** Idle or empty time can be dangerous during the initial quitting process. Stay active and busy.

- **Occupy your hands with other objects.** Use pencils, toothpicks, paper clips, rubber bands, and so on to occupy your hands when you feel something is missing without a cigarette.

- **Beware of cigarette advertisements.** As a smoker you have probably been bombarded with magazine and billboard ads showing healthy, young, attractive individuals smoking. Don't be tempted. After years of smoking, many smokers would not be able to participate in the vigorous activities that are shown in cigarette ads, nor are they able to breathe in and smell the fresh mountain air that is shown. Cigarette advertisements are successful in luring individuals into smoking by appealing to their perceived vulnerabilities. Everyone wants to be seen as attractive, successful, sexy, and fun. The reality is that by being pulled in by these ads you are risking your life.

- **Tell yourself, "Smoking is no longer an option for me."** Immediately after quitting, you may find yourself looking for excuses to justify smoking. Excuses are easy to find when you are looking for them. However, if you have told yourself that smoking is not an option for you anymore, you will need to find another option when you feel stressed or nervous or are finishing a meal. On your quit date, remind yourself that smoking is no longer an option for you and therefore you must handle whatever situation presents itself to you. This statement will empower you to find alternative coping strategies and effectively use them.

Enlist Social Support for Your Quit Date

- **Use your support systems.** Remind your friends and family that you are going through the quitting process and that it is important to you that they support you. Smokers who have more social support have more success in quitting.

- **Be assertive and direct when asking for support.** Everyone needs encouragement and praise for accomplishing and persevering through the difficult process of quitting smoking. Don't view this as a sign of weakness.

- **Negotiate with a live-in smoker.** Living with a smoker may make your efforts to quit smoking more difficult. Therefore, it is important to work out an agreement prior to your quit date that you can both feel comfortable with. For example, you may request that the smoker not leave cigarettes lying around the house.

- **Negotiate with co-workers who smoke.** It is much easier to negotiate with a family member or friend than it is with a co-worker, because loved ones presumably have your best interest at heart. However, this may not be the case with fellow employees. It is important to make a request for support or, at the very least, respect for your efforts to quit smoking. Monitor your own behavior and mood. Get distance from a situation if you feel yourself getting irritated. This will help reduce any potential conflict in the workplace. Finally, you may also need to discuss the office smoking policy with your employer. Be aware of your rights.

Your Quit Date and the Weeks That Follow

- **Pay attention to your high-risk situations.** You are most at risk for *automatically* falling back into your routine of smoking during the first couple of weeks after you quit if you are not vigilant about your high-risk areas. Try to either avoid these situations or at the very least have alternative strategies available.

• **Use distraction techniques.** When you find yourself tempted to smoke a cigarette, get some distance from the thought or situation. Distraction is a wonderful technique to prevent impulsive smoking. This might include physically removing yourself from the situation, shifting your thought to something other than smoking, or engaging in an activity that makes smoking difficult (for example, washing dishes). It is important to remember that the desire to smoke is generally very brief, usually lasting only seconds. Initially after quitting, you may find that the desire for a cigarette feels fairly strong and that you may desire a cigarette quite frequently. However, with time you'll notice that the strength and frequency of the desire will decrease. So if you distract yourself for a brief period of time, the desire will fade, and over time you will not experience the desire as often. Reward yourself each time you successfully distract yourself from the desire.

• **Reinforce your reasons for needing to quit smoking.** During the initial weeks after quitting smoking, you will need to continue reinforcing for yourself your reasons for quitting smoking. Remember that these reasons need to be specific and personal to you. These reasons will help get you through the periods of temptation.

• **Repeat to yourself the benefits of quitting smoking.** You need to remind yourself that good will come of the discomfort, inconvenience, lifestyle changes, and general effort that you are making during this quitting process. Repeat the following list of benefits to yourself several times a day.

Benefits of Quitting Smoking

• Improved circulation

• Decreases or cures allergies (smokers have three times more allergies than nonsmokers)

• Eliminates chronic bronchitis (which decreases energy level, resistance to infection, and predisposes one to emphysema) within a few months after cessation

• Reduces number of cavities and increases chance of keeping your own teeth (smokers have three times more cavities and gum disease than nonsmokers)

• Decreases risk of esophageal cancer by 500 percent

- Decreases risk of kidney cancer by 50 percent
- Decreases frequency and intensity of headaches
- Decreases discomfort and other problems associated with menopause
- Decreases risk of osteoporosis
- Increases lung and breathing capacity
- Increases female fertility by 50 percent
- Significantly decreases your risk for lung cancer and emphysema
- Decreases risk of heart disease

Nicotine Substitution Therapy

The use of nicotine replacement products such as the nicotine gum and patch has been studied for their safe use with cardiac patients. The majority of researchers have found no significant side effects or risk factors for use with individuals with cardiac disease—certainly not as many risk factors as continuing to smoke. Keep in mind that smoking has the greatest number of side effects and risk factors for your heart; the nicotine products have nicotine as the only toxic substance, as compared to your cigarettes, which have over four thousand toxic substances. Therefore, the use of a nicotine product may be a useful aid in your efforts to quit smoking even if you have heart disease. Discuss your current medical condition and the use of these products with your physician. Remember that in order for these products to be most effective, they have to be right for you and used in the proper way.

Although quitting smoking can be a difficult process, it is one of the single most important things that you can do for your heart. Keep in mind that quitting smoking is a process that involves personal motivation and commitment. Continue to reinforce to yourself why you need to quit smoking. Stay focused on the reasons you quit smoking in the first place. Repeat your important reasons to yourself every time you think about a cigarette.

In this chapter, we have outlined the most important steps to successfully quitting smoking. If you find that you require more intensive treatment, you can contact an agency within your community. Whatever method you choose, keep in mind that many smokers make several attempts to quit smoking before they actually succeed. Don't get discouraged if this happens to you. Treat each quit attempt as a learning experience that you can draw from the next time you try. Perseverance, commitment, and personal reasons for needing to quit are the keys to success.

11

Other Risk Factors

Hypertension

High blood pressure, also known as *hypertension*, is a serious independent risk factor for heart disease. Your heart and blood vessels form the cardiovascular system, so any problems in one area will affect the other. Blood pressure is the measure of the force of your blood pushing, or pressing, against the walls of your blood vessels as your heart beats (or pumps) and relaxes. When your blood pressure is measured, you are given two different numbers, such as 120/80 (read "120 over 80"). The top number is your *systolic* pressure and refers to the pressure in your arteries when your heart is pumping. The bottom number is your *diastolic* pressure and refers to the pressure in your arteries when your heart is resting. Your blood pressure can change several times throughout the day depending on your activity and stress level (see chapter 15 for a discussion of how blood pressure increases as a response to stress). Other factors such as diet, being overweight, smoking, and family history can contribute to high blood pressure. For example, too much salt in your diet causes your body to retain fluids, which means your heart has to pump harder; the nicotine in cigarette smoke causes your blood vessels to constrict and therefore increases pressure; and if you are overweight, the heart is working harder to supply the extra body mass.

If you have high blood pressure, this means that your heart has to work harder to handle the higher pressure of the blood against your arteries. In addition, when blood pressure is chronically high, the walls of your arteries become weakened, which then traps the cholesterol and fats as they travel by. Over time, this causes a buildup of fatty plaques which, in turn, narrows the arteries. The heart then has to work harder to pump blood through the clogged arteries. High blood pressure can also cause your arteries to bulge (an *aneurysm*) or burst (a *hemorrhage*).

High blood pressure is defined as blood pressure greater than 140/90 that consistently fails to decrease over a period of time. You may be asked to monitor your blood pressure at different times during the day, as some people have artificially high blood pressure readings because they may be nervous when they are in the doctor's office (this condition is referred to as *white coat hypertension*). Refer to the following table to see where your blood pressure falls:

Table 11.1 Blood Pressure Readings		
	Systolic (upper number) in mm/Hg	Diastolic (lower number) in mm/Hg
Normal	less than 130	less than 85
Borderline	130–139	85–89
Mild High BP	140–159	90–99
Moderate High BP	160–179	100–109
Severe High BP	180–209	110–119
Very Severe High BP	210 or above	120 or above

You should have your blood pressure monitored regularly—at least once per year if you have normal pressure, and every few months if your pressure is borderline or high. Unfortunately, many people receive their first warning of high blood pressure when they suffer a heart attack, stroke, or some other serious problem. The treatment for high blood pressure involves medications (outlined at the end of chapter 3), healthy eating, and other lifestyle changes, such as quitting smoking, exercising regularly, maintaining a healthy weight, and managing your stress in better ways. In short, most of the lifestyle changes discussed in this book will help you keep your blood pressure under control.

Diabetes Mellitus

Approximately fourteen million people in the United States suffer from *diabetes*, a chronic illness that affects the way in which the body produces insulin. *Insulin* is a substance made in the pancreas that regulates how *glucose* (energy) is used by the body. Diabetes is classified according to two types: Type I, or insulin dependent, and Type II, or non-insulin dependent. Insulin-dependent people's bodies produce little or no insulin, and they need to receive insulin injections daily. Non-insulin-dependent people produce insulin, but have difficulty using it efficiently. People with this condition can control their diabetes through diet, weight management, and exercise.

Diabetes carries with it several long-term complications, including heart and kidney disease, circulation problems, and vision disturbances. People with diabetes have more fatty plaques in their blood vessels (atherosclerosis) and higher levels of total cholesterol, LDL cholesterol, and triglycerides. In addition, their HDL cholesterol is lower than in people who do not have diabetes. However, there does not appear to be an increased risk for heart disease in diabetics when their cholesterol level is within normal limits (under 200).

Not only can people who have Type II diabetes control their condition through lifestyle changes, but many of the serious complications associated with diabetes can be avoided by monitoring their blood sugar levels and by strict adherence to diet, exercise, and weight management. Dr. Dean Ornish (1990) found that sticking to a healthy diet and exercising were helpful to the diabetics in his program by reducing their need to take daily insulin shots. Managing your diabetes through diet changes and weight loss allows your body to make the necessary adjustments naturally. You'll also avoid the expense and pain of daily insulin shots. Your physician can give you guidelines on how to control your diabetes. The tips presented in chapter 8 will help you control your cholesterol and lose weight. Exercise with caution, under your physician's care. In addition, you can get more information from the American Diabetes Association.

Snoring

Believe it or not, even what you do while you sleep can indicate potential heart problems. If you are a chronic and loud snorer, you may be more likely to have problems with heart disease. A disorder known as *sleep apnea* has also been associated with increased rates of heart disease, heart attacks, or sudden cardiac death. Sleep apnea is a condition characterized by repeated, periodic interruptions or obstructions of breathing during sleep. If you snore loudly and have periods during which you seem to stop breathing, followed by a noisy return to snoring, then you may have sleep apnea. People with this problem often report feeling sleepy during the daytime, because sleep is continually interrupted by obstructions in breathing. This condition must be diagnosed by a doctor after a careful physical exam.

Snoring, and especially the more severe sleep apnea, can lead to reduced concentrations of oxygen in the bloodstream. The body's response to this often includes elevations in blood pressure and release of stress hormones in the blood. If this happens repeatedly over a long period of time, then it may lead to conditions that are damaging to the heart.

Factors like smoking, alcohol consumption, and obesity make it more likely that you will snore. The actual relationship between snoring (or sleep apnea) and heart disease hasn't been completely clarified yet. It may be that the body's responses to snoring over long periods of time can directly lead to heart difficulties. On the other hand, snoring may not cause cardiac problems directly, but it may serve as an indicator for heart disease because it reflects other risks such as smoking and obesity. Additional research is needed before any conclusions can be drawn. But keep in mind that snoring may indicate more extensive problems than just an unhappy bed partner.

PART 4

Lifestyle Management: Emotional Risk Factors

"Worry is like a rocking chair—it gives you something to do, but it doesn't get you anywhere."

—Dorothy Galyean

12

Dealing with
Depression

Depression has been found to be a significant risk factor for heart disease. So, when you are experiencing emotional pain, your heart may very well be "breaking." The rate of depression among patients with heart disease is strikingly high, at approximately 20 to 30 percent compared to 2 percent among individuals who are not medically ill. Although many cardiac patients and, unfortunately, some of their physicians frequently dismiss or minimize the effects of depression, it is a serious risk factor and complication for cardiac patients. Recent studies have shown that even moderate depression raised the rate of heart disease caused by obstructed coronary arteries by 60 percent and increased the rate of heart attacks by 50 percent (Frasure-Smith, Lesperance, and Talajic 1993). Although smoking, drinking, poor nutrition, and lack of exercise are important risk factors for cardiac disease, when the researchers removed these factors from the equation, depression was the only remaining factor that contributed to this significant increase in heart attacks.

Unfortunately, the word *depression* has been overused and misused by society and therefore has lead to much confusion about what it actually means. For example, it can be used to refer to a mild annoyance: "I'm depressed because I can't get tickets to the baseball game," or to feelings that indicate major clinical depression: "There is no hope, therefore life isn't worth living anymore."

Normal sadness or depression about a specific event or situation is referred to as an *adjustment reaction with a depressed mood*. This type of sadness and depression can occur after a major change or stressor in your life, such as after heart surgery or a heart attack. Although adjustment to many medical conditions can cause depression, cardiac disease can cause intense fears related to the life-threatening nature of the illness and the recurring fear of having another attack. As a result, depression can be quite intense and last for an extended period of time. In addition, changes related to your medical condition such as your possible inability to work and restrictions that may be placed on your personal life can further contribute to the depression. This type of adjustment depression is normal and usually will last for approximately six months after the stressful situation has been resolved. However, the six-month time frame is not set in concrete; it can vary from person to person. Oftentimes when a person is adjusting to a major medical condition and the related financial, emotional, and lifestyle changes that go along with it, the adjustment period can continue for quite some time.

When thinking about depression related to your heart disease, it may be useful to view it as a continuous state with periods of greater intensity when a major change or stressor occurs, like a setback in your medical condition or other personal stressors. This is not to say that depression will be with you forever, but rather that you need to recognize depression in yourself so that it can be successfully treated. Untreated depression puts your heart at further risk for another heart attack and/or complications to your heart disease. Successful identification and treatment of your depression, even if you view it as only moderately severe, can significantly reduce your risk for early death.

From a clinical standpoint, the word *depression* is used to describe negative emotions that can interfere with your relationships, your ability to enjoy life, and your physical health. Many people believe that depression is only about feeling sad and that if they are not sad then they must not be depressed. However, you can feel irritable, anxious, or just plain disinterested with many parts of your life while suffering from depression.

Depressed people often report feeling that activities, events, and people in their lives that used to make them happy no longer do. As a result, many depressed people feel that life is not worth living anymore; some attempt to take their own lives, while others simply stop taking care of themselves. Many cardiac patients who are depressed admit to feeling that following their diet, taking their medication, and regularly following up with their medical appointments is not as important to them as it used to be. They appear to adopt an attitude of "Why bother?" or "What is the point?" Patients who are depressed can also experience difficulty with memory, which frequently interferes with their ability to follow the medical plans their doctors have set up for them.

The following questionnaire was designed to help you recognize symptoms of depression you may be struggling with. It is based on the *DSM*-IV (*Diagnostic and Statistical Manual of Mental Disorders*, fourth edition), which is the diagnostic manual used by mental health professionals.

1. Have you experienced a depressed mood nearly every day for the past several weeks?

2. Have you noticed in the past several weeks that activities, people, or situations that used to give you pleasure no longer interest you in the same way?

3. Have you experienced significant weight loss or weight gain without intentionally trying to change your weight?

4. Are you having difficulty falling asleep and staying asleep at night?

5. Do you find yourself sleeping a lot more than usual?

6. Have other people noticed that you are more restless and agitated than usual?

7. Have other people noticed that you seem more withdrawn?

8. Do you feel more fatigued than usual?

9. Do you feel worthless almost every day?

10. Do you feel guilty almost every day?

11. Do you find that it is harder than it used to be for you to concentrate and make decisions?

12. Do you frequently think about taking your own life?

13. Do you feel that life is not worth living?

14. Do you feel that there is no hope for things to be better?

15. Do you usually feel worse first thing in the morning and therefore find it hard to get out of bed?

If you answered yes to at least five of the questions, including both questions number 1 and 2, and you feel that these symptoms are significantly different from what is "normal" for you and they have significantly impaired your ability to function effectively, then you may be experiencing significant depression.

If you answered yes to some of these questions but not enough to suggest a significant depression, then you may be experiencing a mild type of depression. Perhaps this depressed mood is in response to a particular stressor or because your coping strategies are not particularly effective.

What Does Depression Feel Like to You?

The first step in treating depression is to better identify what *kind* of depression you are experiencing so that you can develop more adaptive strategies to manage it. Symptoms of depression can vary, depending on the individual, and can change at different times. Read through each of the different ways that people experience symptoms of depression and try to identify which "style" is most consistent with your depressive symptoms, either associated with your heart attack or during any low point in your life that you can recall. Place a check mark next to all those symptoms that apply to you during times of depression:

Physically Ill Style

_____ Multiple body aches and pains

_____ Frequent headaches

_____ Poor energy

_____ Stomachache

_____ Poor concentration

_____ Poor memory

_____ Poor appetite

_____ Nausea

_____ Increase in pain that you've had in the past

Anxious Style

_____ Feel like you are "jumping out of your skin"

_____ No interest in doing activities

_____ Feel an extra internal energy, but no desire to act on it

_____ Worry a lot

_____ Feel irritable

_____ Can't sit still

_____ Trouble concentrating on a book or television program

Isolated Style

_____ Want to sleep a lot

_____ Lose interest in interacting with others

_____ Want to be left alone

_____ Not interested in talking to anyone

_____ Frequently call in sick from work

_____ Feel irritated when loved ones inquire about how you are feeling

Dependent Style

_____ Feel insecure

_____ Feel dependent on others to satisfy your needs

_____ Have a chronic knot in your stomach

_____ Cry easily and frequently

_____ Want others around all of the time

_____ Feel frightened most of the time

Were you able to identify with one or more of these styles of depression? Where did the majority of your check marks cluster? In the past, you may not have identified these symptoms as being related to depression but rather to your medical condition or some other stressor. Or, you may have labeled these symptoms as something other than depression. This is usually because, as you can see from the different styles of depression, many of these symptoms can be similar to symptoms related to your medical condition. That makes depression a complex condition to diagnose and treat in the medical patient. However, as you will come to appreciate, it's important to be diagnosed and treated because of the implications it has for your cardiac health.

It is quite common for patients with cardiac disease to struggle to identify which are symptoms of depression and which are symptoms of their disease. Although many symptoms of depression are shared with your medical condition, some are unique to depression (see figure 12.1). Recall your identified style of depression. Once you become comfortable at recognizing your unique symptoms of depression, you'll be in a better position to catch it early on, before it becomes severe. You'll also be better at figuring out which symptoms are unique to your depression and which are part of your cardiac disease. Depression can exacerbate shared symptoms and make them more difficult to manage; therefore, it's important to treat your depression not only to help you feel better emotionally but to improve your physical functioning and overall quality of life.

Hopelessness

Hopelessness is a feeling of despair with no anticipation that the future will be better. Hopelessness also refers to the belief that a situation is not solvable or curable. People who feel hopeless lack self-confidence to solve a problem and are unable to ask others for help because they believe there is no point.

The belief that nothing can ever be better in your life or that you no longer have control over your body or emotional self are two important symptoms of depression that have been linked with cardiac disease. However, although hopelessness can be a symptom of depression, you may feel hopeless and not be suffering from depression.

Studies have shown that people who felt hopeless about the future but were not depressed were more likely to suffer a heart attack than people who maintained their hope, even in those who had no history of angina or prior heart attack (Everson, Goldberg et al. 1996). Therefore, it's important to understand that hopelessness can affect you both psychologically and physically. Psychologically, hopelessness serves to undermine your ability to effectively cope as you adopt a belief that nothing can be better. The situation may seem permanent, and you believe you are too weak and inept to change it. On a physical level, it appears that this feeling of hopelessness may actually influence the immune and nervous system by releasing certain chemicals in the body.

How then do you maintain your hope despite facing serious medical concerns and stressors? The answer lies in how you assess a situation and what you identify as the goal for improvement. For example, living with heart disease can be viewed as a life sentence that limits your ability for happiness. As a result, if your goal is to have no restrictions or changes to your life, then you set yourself up to continue to feel hopeless, as this goal is not realistic. On the other hand, if you view your heart disease as a wake-up call to make important lifestyle changes, you may feel more hopeful about your ability to accomplish that goal and successfully alter your future health.

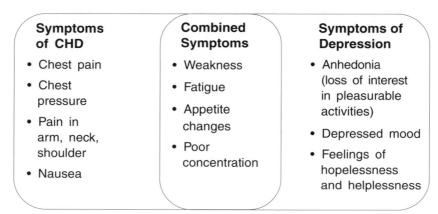

Figure 12.1   Symptoms of Depression and Coronary Heart Disease

Pessimism

Pessimism is a belief that the bad in the world outweighs the good, making this the worst possible of all worlds. A person who is pessimistic tends to take the gloomiest possible view of a situation. Although we have all been pessimistic about particular situations or events, when a pessimistic *style* is adopted it can be harmful to your health.

You may be sitting there reading this and thinking, "I'm not *really* pessimistic because I don't go through life saying to myself that this is the worst of all worlds." While that may be true, pessimistic views can be subtle but still convey the same belief. To help you more clearly identify possible pessimistic views that you hold, read the following questions and place a check mark next to the statement that most typically applies to you.

After you are in a car accident, what are you most likely to say to yourself?

　a. *I'm a terrible driver.*

　b. *I was distracted and not paying attention.*

Following an argument with your spouse, what are you most likely to say to yourself?

　a. *We never get along.*

　b. *We were both tired and irritable.*

After receiving a promotion at work, what are you most likely to say to yourself?

　a. *I was in the right place at the right time and simply got lucky.*

　b. *I've worked very hard and am qualified for this position.*

After you receive a compliment on your appearance, what are you most likely to say to yourself?

　a. *It isn't really me, it's the clothes.*

　b. *I've been working out to get myself in shape.*

When feeling anxious about speaking in front of a crowd, what are you most likely to say to yourself?

　a. *I'm a lousy speaker and shouldn't be asked to speak.*

　b. *I'm anxious because this is a larger crowd than I'm used to addressing.*

When confronted with your cardiac disease, what are you most likely to say to yourself?

　a. *My whole life is over.*

b. *I'm worried about my heart disease but I plan to make many healthy lifestyle changes that will improve the quality of my life.*

When thinking about the cause of your cardiac disease, what are you most likely to say to yourself?

a. *It's my fault and I deserve whatever happens to me.*

b. *I have some responsibility for my heart disease (poor diet, stressful life-style) but I also have genetic risk factors that are beyond my control.*

Did you have more *a* responses than *b* responses? If so, you have a tendency to be more pessimistic than optimistic in your beliefs. Which situations are you more pessimistic about? Are they situations that involve a negative or positive event?

When a bad or stressful event occurs, pessimists are likely to view the cause and result of the event as permanent, believing that the consequences will last forever. Through the eyes of pessimists, everything looks gloomy and is thought of in extreme terms. For example, if they have a problem at work or develop heart disease, then *everything* in their lives is bad. They tend to blame themselves completely for the event, believing that they are a failure. Even when something good occurs, pessimists tend to discount it or attribute it to something or someone else. For example, if a pessimist gets a positive test result back from the doctor, she may believe that the improvement is so minor that it will not have a major impact on her medical condition.

In contrast, optimists view situations and events as isolated. They are able to stay focused on the current event without engaging in extreme thinking. For example, an optimist does not take one setback in his medical disease and generalize it to his whole life. Optimists have confidence in their abilities and believe that they have control over making changes in their lives.

You may be wondering why all of this talk about pessimism and optimism is important in a book about cardiac health. The reason is that having a pessimistic attitude can have a negative impact on your health. For example, you might adopt negative behavior patterns like avoiding necessary health care or isolating yourself from emotional support because you don't trust others. Pessimistic views can immobilize you and therefore prevent you from effectively coping with stressful events. There even appears to be some evidence to suggest that by feeding into your depression, pessimism can indirectly affect your immune system, leaving you too weak to fight off diseases.

Some astounding results from a Canadian study that examined two hundred patients who had recently suffered a heart attack more clearly demonstrates the negative effect pessimism has on cardiac health (Linden, Stossel, and Maurice 1996). The researchers found that the presence of pessimism predicted death *as well as* indicated prior heart attacks and poor heart functioning. When trying to predict death, the level of pessimism of the patient told *more* of the story than artery blockage, cholesterol, high blood pressure, or damage to the heart muscle. After eight years, twenty-one of the twenty-five pessimistic patients were dead in comparison to only six of the twenty-five optimistic patients. This proves that your emotional state can not only leave you *feeling* bad but can also be harmful to your health. Therefore, it's important to aggressively examine and treat feelings of depression in much the same way that you would want your blood pressure to be treated.

How to Manage and Treat Depression

Despite the overwhelming evidence that depression significantly affects your emotional and physical health, are you still thinking, "But it's only depression. I can handle it"? Or, "If I just pull myself together, I can manage this depression"? Or you may be thinking, "Only weak people need to seek out treatment for depression. What do I have to be depressed about? I'm still alive."

When your doctor instructs you to take your heart medicine or medicine for your high blood pressure, do you respond by saying, "I'm strong enough to handle it on my own"? Probably not. Depression is a clinical disorder and should be viewed with the same level of seriousness as your heart disease. It has nothing to do with your character. You may even be trying to justify your feelings of depression, as if you need to find a serious enough reason to give yourself permission to be depressed.

Patients with major depression typically admit to having lost hope, direction, and even the energy to work at making things better. If you've been struggling with depression, you know that at times even minor setbacks with your medical condition or personal life can easily leave you feeling overwhelmed and discouraged. Therefore, when beginning to examine and work on contributing factors to your depression, you need to be specific. The way to manage your depression is to establish goals that can be broken down into subgoals. The use of subgoals allows you to experience a sense of accomplishment, which serves to increase motivation, rally energy, and increase feelings of hope and confidence. In addition, these goals should be personally relevant to you. For example, a specific goal may be to make it through dinner without intrusive thoughts or worries about your heart, or it may be to increase your social interactions with others. To begin formulating goals for managing your depression, answer the following questions about the impact depression is having on your life and what is most important to improve:

What would be better in your life if you were not depressed? ____

What triggers your depression? ____

What makes already existing depression worse? ____

How does your depression interfere with your personal relationships?
____

How does your depression interfere with your medical condition?
____

How do you define a good quality of life? ____

How can you *redefine* your quality of life in light of your medical
limitations? ____

Fight Your Fatigue

Patients with cardiac disease frequently complain of feeling fatigued as part of their medical condition. But fatigue and lack of interest in activities can also be symptoms of depression. Constant fatigue can leave you feeling disinterested in participating in your medical care. It can also leave you without the motivation to make the necessary lifestyle changes that will improve your cardiac health. Let's face it: when you feel chronically tired, you are less likely to be motivated to take good physical and emotional care of yourself. You are also more likely to isolate yourself and avoid pleasurable activities. These behaviors make depression worse. Therefore, symptoms of fatigue should not be ignored. Use the fatigue assessment below to more fully evaluate the role of emotional factors on your energy level.

Fatigue Assessment

What does fatigue and low energy feel like to you? ____

What seems to make the fatigue worse? ____

What seems to make it better? ____

How does fatigue interfere with your day-to-day activities? _____

How does fatigue influence your mood? _____

How do others respond to your low energy? _____

How does your fatigue make you feel about yourself? _____

Techniques to Manage Fatigue

- **Give yourself a break.** When you are under a lot of physical and emotional stress, it's important to take some time and actively withdraw from various activities, decisions, and conflicts. This slowing-down period should be viewed as an opportunity for you to recharge your battery. Give yourself permission to withdraw for a while while you focus on what you need to do to improve your motivation to make healthy changes. This withdrawal time should be viewed as temporary and not as an opportunity to isolate yourself.

- **Focus on what's important and let the rest go.** Take your time to evaluate the situation *and* your resources to cope. You do not have to impulsively jump into every stressful event with both feet. Next, apply your coping skills. For example, when confronted with the need for an angioplasty procedure, don't avoid the decision by dwelling on a minor detail about scheduling. This only burns up your energy with no productive gain. Rather, step back and allow yourself time to emotionally and intellectually process the information and *then* decide which coping skills will work best for you during the procedure—for example, the distraction techniques or actively seeking information about the procedure. By focusing on what's important to you, you actually feel more energized and prepared to deal with the procedure.

- **Learn to take time just for yourself.** Does this concept sound foreign? Oftentimes when our lives become hectic and regimented we lose sight of the importance of taking time to take care of ourselves. We write it off as "frivolous," "wasted energy," or "unnecessary." We dismiss the idea because it makes us feel selfish or needy. Do you have reservations or fears about taking time for yourself? The most important thing you can do to manage your fatigue is to take time to care for yourself. Your medical condition, stressors in your life, and depression can leave you depleted of energy that is essential for your emotional and physical health. Following is a list of some possible ways to escape or withdraw during particularly stressful times:

- Take hot showers or baths

- Meditate

- Read

- Take long walks or drives

- Use relaxation techniques (see chapter 15)

Cope with Feelings of Loss and Change

If you have cardiac disease, the magnitude of loss and change is significant for you because it involves multiple areas of your life. These areas can include

- How you view your body

- Fears about how others will view you (as weak or fragile)

- Your ability to work in the same capacity as before

- Loss of security about your health and future

- Diet

- Establishing exercise programs

- Learning new techniques for managing feelings and conflicts

- Fears about the impact your heart disease will have on your sex life

When you develop a major illness like cardiac disease or have suffered a heart attack, it's easy to begin feeling vulnerable about the changes in your life. This can lead to feelings of hopelessness, which can not only worsen depression, but can actually increase the risk of suffering a heart attack. Learning strategies to remain hopeful and less depressed about the changes and related losses in your life is a way of improving your health. The following strategies can help you manage feelings of hopelessness and loss associated with changes in your life after a heart attack.

- **Establish realistic expectations.** Acknowledge that there will be changes in your life as a result of your heart disease. Patients who hope for life to be exactly the way it was before set themselves up for disappointment. Use the following questions to more fully examine your expectations:

What are your expectations in terms of how your medical condition will affect you? _____

_____

_____

Do you expect to be cured? _____

How do you envision life after a heart attack? _____

_____

_____

What do you expect from your doctors? _____

_____

_____

What do you expect from your family? _____

_____

_____

Do you believe that your illness is a punishment from God and therefore something out of your control? _____

Do you view yourself as an unlucky person? _____

Do you expect that you will be unable to make changes in your life? _____

Do you believe that your cardiac disease will negatively affect your personal relationships? _____

Review your answers. Are they realistic? Do you have enough information to answer the questions? If not, then seek out medical guidance and talk to significant others in your life to prevent having false expectations.

- **When attempting to cope or change a stressor, begin by breaking the situation down into workable pieces.** For example, when looking at the lifestyle changes you need to make, break them down one at a time. Examine your diet, make basic changes first, and then begin to experiment with recipes and ways to substitute healthy ingredients in your favorite recipes. With each small change you make, you'll feel more confident in your abilities and more hopeful about your health.

- **Take control over things that are within your control and let go of wasting energy on things that you can't change.** A normal reaction to living with cardiac disease is to feel a loss of control over your life. Evaluate which things you do have control over and exercise that control. For example, you have control over improving your cardiac health by making certain lifestyle changes. Monitor any negative statements you may be making to yourself, such as, "Nothing I can do will make a difference. If I'm going to suffer another heart attack it's just going to happen." Use the following checklists to assess what makes you feel out of control and dependent.

Physical Changes

_____ Significant weight loss

_____ Scars from surgical incisions

_____ Weakness

_____ Fatigue

_____ Sexual changes

_____ Headaches

_____ Nausea

_____ Increased medications

_____ Changes in diet

_____ Difficulty sleeping

_____ Other _____

Psychosocial Changes

_____ Loss of job

_____ Can only work in part-time jobs

_____ Loss of financial security

_____ Unable to be as physically active as in the past

_____ More dependent on others

_____ Feelings of helplessness

_____ Feelings of anxiety and fear

_____ Irritability

_____ Loss of control over your schedule

_____ Family having problems coping with your illness

_____ Marital problems

_____ Can't parent your children the way you would like

_____ Don't feel as masculine anymore

_____ Don't feel as feminine anymore

_____ Afraid that your loved one will leave you

_____ Loss of personal freedom with multiple hospitalizations

_____ Awareness of the reality of decreased life expectancy

_____ Other _____

Once you've identified the changes that make you feel most out of control, begin to monitor what you say to yourself about these changes and what you fear others are thinking about regarding these changes. Practice substituting realistic and healthy coping statements for each of these changes. For example, "I feel more dependent on others" becomes "It's healthy for me to rely on others to help me through this stressful time."

Medications for Treatment of Depression in Cardiac Patients

Approximately 65 to 80 percent of patients with major depression are effectively treated with antidepressant medications (Rand 1991). The goal in treating depression with an antidepressant medication is to effectively improve the depression while minimizing any side effects or safety concerns. As a patient with cardiac disease, you may be worrying about which drugs are safest for you. This is an important question that you should discuss with your doctor. Don't avoid the issue of talking about the possibility of using an antidepressant because of fear of side effects. Remember, one of the worst things you can do for your heart is to leave depression untreated.

There are four primary classes or types of antidepressants. These include the selective serotonin reuptake inhibitors (SSRIs), tricyclic antidepressants (TCAs), monoamine oxidase inhibitors (MAOIs) and atypical antidepressants. Each type of drug has strengths and weakness in terms of side effects and safety.

SSRIs

These represent a relatively new class of antidepressant that works by increasing the amount of serotonin in the brain. Some SSRIs are sertraline (Zoloft), fluoxetine (Prozac), and paroxetine (Paxil). As a group of medications, SSRIs are as effective as other antidepressants without as many side effects for the cardiac patient. The rate of discontinuation of these drugs due to problematic side effects is lower than with other antidepressants. It has been recommended that SSRIs be the first choice of antidepressant for patients with cardiac disease. The side effects associated with the SSRIs include nausea, diarrhea, anxiety or jittery feeling and insomnia. Men may also experience delayed ejaculation or impotence and women may experience anorgasmia, or the inability to have an orgasm.

TCAs

These include amitriptyline (Elavil), doxepin (Sinequan), imipramine (Tofranil), and nortriptyline (Pamelor), and are not the first choice of drugs for patients with cardiac disease. They are associated with a number of cardiotoxic effects. In addition, they are also associated with decrease in blood pressure when you stand up, sedation, dry mouth, blurred vision, constipation, an inability to urinate, and sexual dysfunction. Some of the TCAs have been used to help nondepressed patients sleep because they are so sedating. However, as a cardiac patient you need to talk to your doctor about potential side effects and complications of using a TCA.

MAOIs

These drugs were originally used as antituberculosis medications. Approximately forty years ago, it was observed that patients who were on these drugs experienced mood elevations. The MAOIs were then discovered to be useful as antidepressants. Medications in this class include tranylcypromine (Parnate), phenelzine (Nardil), and isocarboxazid (Marplan). Two major limiting factors in using these drugs is that they are not as effective as other antidepressants, and patients must significantly alter their diets to avoid serious side effects. The diet must be low in tyramine, which means patients must avoid aged cheeses, red wines, chocolate, beer, smoked fish, liver, dry sausage, and fava beans. Certain medications should also be avoided.

Other Antidepressants

Some antidepressant medications do not fit in any of the typical categories. These drugs include bupropion (Wellbutrin), trazadone (Desyrel), nefazodone (Serzone), and venlafaxine (Effexor).

Wellbutrin is recommended as the second choice of medication for depression in cardiac patients who experience intolerable side effects to the SSRIs, such as sexual dysfunction. It has very few cardiovascular side effects and does not cause side effects such as constipation, indigestion, nausea, and so on. It also does *not* cause your blood pressure to drop when you stand up. In studies that have compared the effectiveness of Wellbutrin in treating moderate to severe depression to that of the TCAs and SSRIs, it has been found to be equally as effective (Feighner, Gardner, Johnston et al. 1991).

Desyrel has been found to be as effective as the TCAs but causes sedation and can cause your blood pressure to drop when you stand up. Further, it has also been associated with arrhythmias in cardiac patients.

Serzone is similar in its chemical properties to Desyrel but does not have as many side effects. It has very few cardiotoxic effects. The main side effects include dizziness, nausea, dry mouth, sedation, and weakness.

Effexor is a relatively new antidepressant on the market. Clinically, it has been proven to be effective with patients who suffer from depression that has not improved with other medications. Chemically, it is unrelated to any other antidepressant. The main problem or side effect with this drug appears to be that it leads to an increase in blood pressure that tends to remain elevated. Although some studies have suggested that the blood pressure increase is related to the dose of the medication (Montgomery 1993), as a cardiac patient this would not be the first choice of antidepressant.

Summary of Strategies for Beating Depression

Have you been able to recognize depressive symptoms in yourself and how they may be interfering in your recovery process? Hopefully, this chapter on depression has convinced you that depression needs to be recognized early and treated aggressively.

Although we have outlined psychological strategies for you to work through on your own, we strongly encourage you to seek out professional help if your mood does not improve. Also, it's important to stay open-minded and discuss with your physician the pros and cons of using an antidepressant medication. Review the following strategies whenever you feel depression coming on:

- Recognize your depression triggers.

- Avoid isolating yourself. Social isolation reinforces feelings of despair and has been identified as a major risk factor for cardiac disease.

- Push yourself to engage in small tasks. Lack of engagment in activities or life in general leads to decreased energy and increased depression. Feelings of fatigue may well be a combination of your medical condition and depression. Take control over this symptom by engaging in small and reasonable activities.

- Take time to care for yourself. Renew your energy and your ability to stay healthy by doing pleasurable things for yourself.

- Get support from others.

- Practice making optimistic and realistic statements to yourself.

- Avoid thinking in extremes. For example, "*Everything* is terrible in my life because I have cardiac disease."

- Objectively evaluate what you can control. Break controllable items into workable goals and let go of those things over which you have no control.

- Remember, depression is a significant risk factor for heart disease. Take care of your heart by effectively treating your depression. Make it as important as treating your blood pressure or your diet.

- Seek professional help when needed.

- Consult with your physician on the benefits and risks of an antidepressant medication.

13

Social Isolation

Being alone or socially isolated can not only leave you feeling sad and distressed but can also be harmful to your heart. Many studies have shown that having strong support from friends and family members can help to keep your blood pressure down and your heart functioning well. Uchino and Cacioppo (1996) found that when subjects were performing a stressful act, they were able to keep their heart rates lower when they were with a friend as opposed to a stranger.

Research has also shown that you are more at risk to die after a heart attack if you live alone. It's unclear if this is because people who feel isolated and alone are more depressed and therefore give up on living by not taking their medications, following their diets, and so on. Whatever the reason may be, it's clear that feeling lonely and unsupported by others is a contributing factor to early death. In Uchino and Cacioppo's 1996 study of thirteen hundred people with heart disease, 82 percent of them who had someone that they could confide in about their feelings and physical condition were still alive after five years. However, only 50 percent of those who were isolated and without a confidant were still alive after five years.

Are You Socially Isolated?

Researchers have identified several factors that define social isolation. Answering the following questions about yourself will help you discover if these factors are present in your life. Keep in mind that it is normal and, at times, healthy to have periods of isolation. For example, immediately after a stressful event it may be both necessary and healthy to withdraw into yourself. However, the concept of social isolation involves a chronic pattern. Therefore, when answering the following questions, consider what a usual pattern for you might be.

Are you someone who tends to keep feelings to yourself? _____

Have you avoided openly communicating with your doctors about your medical condition? _____

Do you have many friends and family members but don't *feel* supported? _____

Do you avoid organized churches or groups? _____

Do you feel as though you have no one to turn to when you have a problem? _____

Do you feel as though you have no one to rely on to help you make decisions? _____

If you answered yes to three or more of the questions, then you may be increasing your risk for an early death. Research has shown that people who are socially isolated or who *feel* that they lack support from others were twice as likely to die of heart disease than those who had positive social support (Uchino and Cacioppo 1996).

Social Support

Social support can be defined in tangible and measurable ways such as the number of friends or personal relationships you have. It can also be defined in more subjective ways, such as the *feeling* of being connected to others. However the concept of social support is defined, there is substantial evidence that it has direct effects on psychological and physical well-being as well as indirect stress-buffering effects (Cohen and Wills 1985). Having a poor social support system has been identified as a major risk factor for depression, suicide, and heart disease.

House (1981) has defined social support as consisting of four different types of support: emotional, instrumental, informational, and appraisal. *Emotional support* includes receiving expressions of love, empathy, trust, and genuine caring. *Instrumental support* provides the individual with direct services that are tangible. *Informational support* involves providing advice, suggestions, and information to influence the thoughts and behaviors of others. *Appraisal support* includes constructive feedback, affirmation, and social comparison information that allows the individual to engage in self-evaluation.

Just as there are a variety of ways to conceptualize and define social support, there are also a variety of personal styles and needs regarding social support. Social support can mean different things to different people. For example, some people find support and comfort in being alone, and others may feel more comfortable with one-on-one support; still others may enjoy the dynamics of a group experience. It's important to identify what kind of support works best for you. To assess your personal needs and comfort level with social support, answer the following questions:

Social Style Questionnaire

1. When you feel sad or down in the dumps, do you tend to want to be alone? _____

2. During periods of sadness or depression, do you feel better when you're around others? _____

3. Do you feel comfortable confiding in just one good friend? _____

4. Does knowing that others are feeling what you're feeling or experiencing what you're experiencing make you feel supported? _____

5. Do you tend to feel awkward in social situations and generally feel uncomfortable in groups? _____

6. Do you find that listening to other people's similar concerns makes you feel worse instead of better? _____

7. Do you cope better with your concerns when you're simply left alone? _____

If you answered yes to questions 1, 5, 6, and 7, you probably tend to cope better when left alone. You might not feel comfortable in a support group or using a buddy system. However, you may benefit from instrumental or informational support. That is, although receiving emotional support may not be valued or important to you, obtaining available resources, such as advice or suggestions, may be useful in providing you with some type of support.

In contrast, if you answered yes to questions 2, 3, and 5, this suggests that you are generally more comfortable confiding in one person or you tend to feel awkward in social groups; you may need to establish a one-on-one support system, or you may need to strengthen a preexisting one.

If you answered yes to questions 2, 3, and 4, then you are quite comfortable in social settings and find comfort in sharing feelings and experiences with others and knowing that they are feeling the same thing; it is appraisal support that you seek, and support groups may be useful for you.

In addition to your social style, the stage of your coping is important to keep in mind, as some types of support are better suited for different stages of coping. For example, if you have just recently been told that you have heart disease or have just recently suffered a heart attack, you may need emotional support. However, as you begin to adjust to new lifestyle changes that are necessary for the health of your heart, you may require more informational or instrumental support. This support may come from consultations with a dietician on how to maintain your heart-healthy diet, or it may include active involvement with a rehabilitation program with exercise training and so on.

It is important to recognize the benefits of having a good social support network of any type. These benefits include

- Improvement in your physical health

- Improvement in your emotional health

- Increased energy and motivation when you feel supported by others

- Opportunity to obtain information about the medical conditions and experiences of others who share similar situation

- Decreased feelings of loneliness and isolation when you feel connected to others

- Decreased risk factor for early death after heart attack

How is your social support network? Remember, it is not only important to examine what support systems you have but also how supported you feel by that system. Answer the following questions to assess your own social system. This will be helpful in identifying potential areas that are weak and in need of improvement. For example, maybe you will discover that you have many people in your life who can provide you with emotional support, but you are lacking in information specific to your medical illness or are feeling disconnected from others who share your same medical illness.

Assess Your Social Support Network

- Whom do you generally rely on for emotional support? _____

- Is this person consistently available to you? _____

- Do you have tangible support (adequate finances, etc.)? _____

- Are you able to recognize when support is needed? _____

- Can you readily access the support system? _____

- Are you connected to extended community networks (support agencies, other cardiac patients)? _____

- Are you able to assertively ask for support? _____

- Do you believe that good social support is essential to physical and emotional well-being? _____

Techniques to Improve Your Social Support

1. Establish what type of social support would be most useful for you, given your social style and current stage of coping. Use the Social Style Questionnaire on page 165.

2. Increase emotional and instrumental support from family or friends by including them in your care. Family members or friends who are well educated about your medical needs and concerns are in a better position to provide emotional support. Also, they can provide instrumental support by becoming more involved in your care—for example, by taking your blood pressure, assisting with medication, and so on.

3. Educate yourself about existing social networks of others who've been through similar situations. Obtain information on community resources and local support groups for cardiac patients. Remind yourself about the advantages of interacting with other cardiac patients who may be experiencing similar concerns. They may be able to provide you with information on strategies they have successfully used in monitoring their diet or other lifestyle changes. You may also benefit from interactions with other cardiac patients by learning that the emotions you're experiencing are shared by others.

4. Learn how to develop a buddy system. A buddy system typically involves two cardiac patients who join forces to support each other with their diet, limitations in physical activities, and changes in lifestyle. Make a list of possible candidates and then examine the advantages and disadvantages of your choices.

5. Learn how to be assertive when asking for support from others. Oftentimes cardiac patients will report not wanting to "be a burden to their family or friends" or to appear to be "whining or complaining all the time." Begin by making a list of what you need from individuals in your support system. Then practice asking for those needs without feeling like a burden or complainer. This can be accomplished by following these steps:

   a. Outline what you need and from whom and then practice more effective communication skills to address these needs. Frequently, family members and friends of chronically ill people do not know what to say or do to be helpful. Finding a balance between helping without making the person totally dependent on them is a struggle for supportive family members and friends. Similarly, you may be struggling with the same issues.

b. Learn the difference between assertiveness and aggressiveness. *Assertiveness* is the balance between two extremes of *aggressiveness* and *submissiveness*. People who act in an aggressive style demand and expect others to do exactly what they want. Those who act in a submissive style give up their own beliefs, opinions, and wants for those of others. They feel guilty asking for what they want, as if others' needs were more important than their own. Assertive people respect others' views and feelings but also value and respect their own.

c. Learn how to be specific when making a request. Vague requests or comments can often be misinterpreted by others or simply ignored. If your request is specific and direct, there is little room for confusion. For example, instead of asking for someone's help in general, state specifically *what* you want help with, *when*, and for *how long*.

14

Understanding
Personality Factors

Your personality defines who you are, how you make decisions, and the way in which you interact with the world. Personality style is an enduring trait that grows out of a combination of childhood experiences and heredity. It remains relatively consistent throughout your life. Your personality style is important because it not only affects your relationships and interactions with others, but it can also affect your health. Certain styles can actually weaken the heart and increase the risk of heart disease. These same styles can also interfere with the potential benefits of a variety of cardiac treatments designed to improve the condition of your heart. The riskiest personality styles for your heart include negative patterns of emotional expression and the "coronary-prone personality," also known as Type A personality or Type A behavior pattern. The components of the Type A pattern that appear most damaging to your heart are

- A hostile, angry approach to life
- A consistent feeling of time pressure

These styles of thinking, feeling, and acting cause problems because they appear to lead to physical changes over time that may damage the heart. In addition, they may increase the likelihood of heart-destructive behaviors, such as smoking, alcohol abuse, poor eating habits, and avoidance of proper medical care.

Type A Personality

Do you know someone who is a pressured overachiever, who never has enough time in the day to accomplish all his or her goals? Someone who is highly competitive, easily annoyed and irritated, with a hostile, surly, even rude demeanor? Someone who never seems to relax or slow down, but is impatient, juggling more than one activity at a time? If you or a loved one have most of these qualities, then chances are, you qualify as having a *coronary-prone*, or *Type A*, personality.

In the 1950s, a group of researchers headed by cardiologists Meyer Friedman and Ray Rosenman were perplexed by the finding that traditional medical risk factors did not seem to explain the full picture of heart disease (Friedman and Ulmer 1984). In fact, up to half of the factors accounting for heart disease seemed to be missing. Then they observed that the majority of their heart patients, who were mostly men, shared common behaviors and styles of interacting. Their patients seemed caught in a constant struggle to achieve more and more in less and less time. Something always seemed to be standing in the way of their attempts, frustrating their efforts to achieve. This frustration was often accompanied by angry, irritable, and hostile demeanors. These patients often exhibited underlying feelings of insecurity, perhaps due to a lack of love, encouragement, and affection when they were young. These components appeared to be interrelated, so that an increase in one led to an increase in the others. The qualities also seemed to be persistent over time. For example, the more insecure they felt, the more frustrated and irritable they became, and subsequently their attitude became hostile.

Drs. Friedman and Rosenman named this pattern the Type A behavior pattern and began exploring its relationship to heart disease. In the past forty years of research in this area, efforts have been made to identify the components of this pattern that are most related to heart disease. Consistently, a feeling of time pressure or impatience and an ever present hostility have been suggested as the most heart-destructive qualities.

The most recent evidence suggests that a hostile approach to life puts you at greatest risk for developing heart disease. The risks associated with living under time pressure have become more controversial. If you have a busy, pressured life, but you meet your challenges with a positive, confident approach, then your risk of heart disease may not be significantly greater. This may reflect the "work hard, play hard" mentality. If you live a balanced life and feel confident and secure in your ability to meet your challenges, then living with a frequent sense of time pressure is probably not as damaging to your heart. Nevertheless, it may lead you to lifestyle patterns that are harmful to your heart. For example, being constantly busy and pressed for time may leave you little time or energy for preparing healthy foods or for exercise. Additionally, you may be prone to engage in bad habits—like smoking, use of drugs or alcohol—for quick fixes to feeling tense, rather than take time for more appropriate ways of managing stress. More details about managing your own levels of time pressure and anger are discussed later in this chapter.

The easiest way to identify Type A behavior is to look for signs of impatience, a sense of time urgency, and an ever present aggressive attitude. The best way to identify the Type A behavior pattern in a person is to have a professional, such as a psychologist, diagnose it after making observations during a structured interview. However, you can get an idea of how many Type A qualities you have by filling out the following questionnaire. You can also rate the presence of these qualities in a loved one. Two parts of the questionnaire are designed to be answered by a significant other, and two are designed to be answered by you. If you have a Type A personality yourself, you may have trouble admitting it. The majority of people with Type A find this status hard to accept or acknowledge in themselves. Therefore, it's important to have a loved one rate you on the physical signs of anger, hostility, and time pressure. Try to keep an open mind and be honest in rating yourself.

The Type A Personality Questionnaire*

Use the following rating system:

1 = Never
2 = Sometimes
3 = Always

Physical Signs of Anger and Hostility

Have a significant other answer these questions.

_____ Does the person's face look hostile?

_____ Does the person usually have a sneer on his or her face?

_____ Is the person's jaw or mouth usually tight?

_____ When the person laughs, is it jarring and hostile?

_____ Does the person usually clench his or her fists during ordinary social conversations?

_____ Does the person have unpleasant, loud, and grating speech?

_____ Does the person frequently use profanity?

_____ Does the person typically grind his or her teeth when awake or during sleep?

---

*Items adapted from Friedman and Ulmer's *Treating Type A Behavior and Your Heart* (1984) and Friedman and Ghandour's "Medical Diagnosis of Type A Behavior" (1993).

Lifestyle Indicators of Anger and Hostility

Answer these questions yourself.

_____ Do you enjoy a fierce, competitive approach to activities?

_____ Do you get frustrated when you lose, even in minor contests or in contests with children?

_____ Are you easily frustrated or annoyed by the incompetence of others?

_____ Do you strongly defend opinions on social, political, or economic issues?

_____ Is it hard for you to feel happy at the success of others?

_____ Do you have difficulty sleeping because of feeling frustrated about events of the day?

_____ Do you feel in competition with, or overly criticized by, your significant other?

Physical Signs of a Sense of Time Pressure

Have a significant other answer these questions.

_____ Does the person usually look tense around the mouth and eyebrows?

_____ Does the person rapidly blink his or her eyes?

_____ Does the person's body look tense, as if he or she is always ready to spring into action?

_____ Does the person typically make hurried, jerky movements?

_____ Does the person often shrug his or her shoulders?

_____ Does the person speak in a rapid manner?

_____ Does the person frequently interrupt others?

_____ Does the person usually attempt to hurry the speech of others?

_____ Does the person often fidget, such as by rapid tapping of fingers or jiggling knees?

_____ Does the person nod his or her head when speaking (as compared to nodding in agreement when others are speaking)?

_____ Does the person have a habit of quickly drawing in a breath while speaking?

_____ Does the person make clicking sounds with his or her lips while speaking?

_____ Does the person have a tendency to move and act quickly?

_____ Does the person repeatedly sigh when exhaling?

Lifestyle Indicators of Time Pressure

Answer these questions yourself.

_____ Do you usually feel in a rush to get things done?

_____ Would you consider yourself impatient?

_____ Do you maintain such a busy pace of life that others frequently advise you to slow down?

_____ Is it hard for you to sit still and do nothing?

_____ Do you become intensely annoyed at waiting in line?

_____ Do you talk and eat quickly?

_____ Do you tend to juggle more than one activity at a time?

_____ Do you tend to think of other things while speaking with someone?

_____ Do you make a point of never being late for appointments?

_____ Do you enjoy reminiscing about old times?

_____ Do you take time out to enjoy things around you, like nature?

Add your total score for the items that were rated by your significant other. Then add your scores from the questions that you rated yourself. There is no cutoff score to indicate Type A personality, however, the more questions that were scored as a 3, and the higher your total overall score, the more likely you are to show the Type A behavior pattern. Also, examine the difference between scores you gave yourself as compared to those ratings by your loved one. You may find that others see more of these behaviors in you than you are willing to acknowledge in yourself.

Type B Personality

In contrast to the Type A personality, are you the relaxed, unhurried type who is not bothered by a sense of time pressure? Rather than regularly experiencing frustration or hostility, do you feel at ease, self-confident, and able to enjoy well-rounded activities and relationships? Then you would be considered more of a Type B person. Type B persons have typically been defined by a lack of Type A characteristics. More importantly, people with Type B characteristics have a significantly lower risk of heart disease than those with Type A behaviors. If you have few or no signs of Type A behavior, then your chances of developing heart disease before age sixty are slim.

Some people (probably those with a lot of Type A qualities) assume that if you are not a hard-driving Type A kind of person, then that means you are lazy and unmotivated. This is not necessarily the case. Though some may be unmotivated, many Type B individuals achieve great success in their careers and other endeavors. They are more successful in juggling their responsibilities without constantly feeling under the gun, pressured, and frustrated. They enjoy a balance in their lives between work and relaxing enjoyment of other activities and relationships.

While some people may fit neatly into either a strong Type A or a clear-cut Type B style, many probably fall somewhere in the middle—having qualities of both. Others may react differently in varying situations. In general, if you are more often and more strongly Type B, you can feel reassured that your approach to life is probably good for your heart. If you are in the middle, you could do better at limiting the times when you are impatient, hostile, or angry. If you are a strong Type A, be aware of the strain you're putting on your heart, your emotional well-being, and your family relationships.

Since most of the research in this area has involved more men than women, you should keep in mind that this description may not apply as much to women. In fact, researchers have observed that Type A women are less likely than Type A men to display socially the verbal and physical signs of time pressure and hostility (Friedman and Ulmer 1984). While Type A women tend to speak rapidly, hurry the speech of others, and seem distracted or preoccupied in social conversations, they are more likely to be frustrated instead of overtly hostile or aggressive in their actions.

How Does Type A Personality Affect Your Health?

In 1980, a National Institutes of Heath panel concluded that Type A behavior is an independent risk factor equal to or greater than other traditional risk factors for heart disease—such as obesity, smoking, diabetes, and high blood pressure (cited in Friedman and Ulmer 1984). Results of studies include the following discoveries:

- Persons with the Type A behavior pattern, whether male or female, are up to seven times more likely to have heart disease than Type B persons.

- Healthy Type A men are two to three times more likely than Type B men to suffer a heart attack.

- A person under sixty years of age who suffers a heart attack almost always shows the Type A behavior pattern.

- Type A behavior is associated with increased levels of cholesterol and triglycerides, high blood pressure, and excess release of insulin after eating sugar.

- Type A behavior has been associated with delays in seeking treatment for symptoms of heart disease, which can greatly reduce effectiveness of medical treatments.

- People with silent ischemia tend to show Type A behavior.

Type A behaviors, specifically hostility, have a negative effect on your body. For example, when you feel angry and hostile over a long period of time, your brain releases a larger amount of stress hormones into your blood. This can lead to greater wear and tear on your blood vessels, making them more likely to constrict and become lined with blockages. Regularly occurring hostility can also cause your blood to become stickier (platelet activation), and this in turn can make blood clots form more easily. Feeling angry and hostile can also lead to an increase in total cholesterol levels. These physiological reactions are related to the body's stress response.

Having a chronically negative, hostile approach to life can also interfere with your response to certain medical treatments. Hostility has been investigated in relation to adjustment after balloon angioplasty procedures. A major difficulty associated with this procedure is the likelihood of *re-stenosis*, or blockage building up again in the treated artery. This happens in about half of treated arteries and may require repeat angioplasty. A recent study found that patients with hostile personalities were two-and-a-half times more likely to have re-stenosis than patients with low hostility (Goodman et al. 1996). This finding, however, was true for white men, but not for women or African-Americans. The majority of women and African-American patients had low ratings for hostility but relatively high rates of re-stenosis. This suggests that other factors—as yet to be determined—are more relevant for these groups.

Type A and Heart Disease

Type A behavior appears to do its damage to the heart through three main avenues:

1. By leading to an increase in traditional risk factors such as smoking, obesity, alcohol abuse, and high blood pressure.

2. By triggering the fight-or-flight response. Your body responds to the stress you perceive on the outside by releasing adrenaline and other stress hormones in order to prepare you

to either face or flee from your challenges. Adrenaline causes heart rate and blood pressure to rise, and platelets in the blood to become stickier. If this happens occasionally in response to temporary challenges, it won't cause significant problems for your health. In fact, it is your body's positive way of assisting you in dealing with the challenges in your life. However, because Type A persons tend to repeatedly feel tense, impatient, and agitated, their fight-or-flight response may be activated on a regular basis. This exposes the heart and blood vessels to chronically high and perhaps damaging levels of stress hormones. As arteries narrow and blood flow decreases, chest pains or heart attacks may result. The fight-or-flight response also causes blood to be directed away from organs such as the liver and toward the heart, brain, and muscles. This may contribute to the increased cholesterol levels found in people with Type A personality: with decreased blood supply, the liver cannot remove or metabolize cholesterol and fat as well.

3. By interfering with seeking appropriate treatment for symptoms of heart disease. Type A persons tend to focus on outside activities instead of on inner bodily experiences. This may lead to a tendency to ignore distress signals from the body or postpone attention to them by focusing on external tasks.

Hot Reactors

Dr. Robert Eliot (1984), a cardiologist who himself suffered a heart attack, identified a group of people at increased risk of heart troubles as *hot reactors*. These are persons who display extreme cardiovascular responses to stressful situations—even those occurring in typical daily life. For example, a hot reactor might experience a large jump in blood pressure when dealing with a traffic jam. Approximately 20 percent of healthy people will be hot reactors under stress, and Type A persons are more likely to show these kinds of reactions. Chronically high levels of anger and hostility may lead people with Type A to have higher resting blood pressure, as well as further spiking of blood pressure when stressed. Holding anger in, especially when combined with a higher resting blood pressure or a family history of hypertension, has been associated with greater increases in blood pressure during mental stress—the hot reactor phenomenon—but interestingly, only for men. Men also tend to show greater elevations in stress hormones and in LDL cholesterol levels in response to lab stresses (Stoney et al. 1988). Some studies have actually shown a positive effect of holding anger in for women. For example, one study indicated that women with anger-in tendencies showed a faster recovery in blood pressure changes associated with an anger-provoking task (Lai and Linden 1992). Women may be more uncomfortable with outward expressions of anger and hostility, and therefore less distressed than men by withholding these feelings. See chapter 16 for further discussion of factors more relevant for women.

Recent studies exploring the hot reactor phenomenon have suggested that persons who overreact to mental stress are up to twenty times more likely to have silent heart disease (Jiang et al. 1996; Margolis 1996). Those with ischemia during mental stress were almost three times more likely to have a cardiac event such as heart attack as patients without ischemia during stress. Overall, these findings suggest that in healthy people, especially those with genetic risk factors, a physiological overresponse to everyday stress may be a new marker for heart disease. Unfortunately, most hot reactors are not aware of the great physical responses they experience under stress. This makes identifying this tendency difficult to do at home. If you have a home blood pressure monitor, comparing blood pressure levels at rest and then during a stressful situation may give you an idea of the differences, which you can then discuss with your doctor. Dr. Eliot also discusses a formula you may use at home that give clues to the presence of hot reacting (you can find information about his book in Appendix B, Further Reading).

Type D Personality

Your particular style of coping with stress may lead to emotional responses that are bad for your health. For instance, if you tend to deny or push aside upsetting feelings on a regular basis, then you are at greater risk for heart disease. This style has been termed the Type D personality, referring to the tendency to deny or hold in distressing feelings. A recent study found that the death rate for Type D heart patients was four times higher than that for patients more open in discussing feelings (Denollet et al. 1996). If you have already had a heart attack and you have this style of dealing with stress, then you may be up to six times more likely to die from heart disease than others who are more open and flexible in dealing with their feelings. Specifically, if you avoid dealing with depressed feelings, you're more likely to develop atherosclerosis (Ketterer et al. 1996). If you deny angry feelings, you may be at greater risk of ischemia and silent ischemia during stress testing as well as in stressful life circumstances. If you have a more general difficulty in identifying and expressing emotions, also known as *alexithymia*, you may be at greater risk of developing atherosclerosis and ignoring symptoms of a heart attack (Kenyon et al. 1991; Ketterer et al. 1991a). This quality is described in more detail in chapter 4.

If you are the type who has trouble identifying or expressing emotions, or you tend to deny upsetting feelings, then it may be hard for you to recognize your own distressed states. Obtaining feedback from loved ones as to how they rate you on qualities such as depression and anger may be helpful. In addition, when you are feeling bad, stop and take time to examine the specifics of what you are feeling. Are you angry, frustrated, insecure, guilty, sad, fatigued? Putting a specific label on your feelings can help you identify what events have contributed to those feelings. It will also make it easier to address the situations that caused you to feel the way you do. If you sweep your worries under the carpet and avoid dealing with them, then the conflicts don't get resolved. They will simply recur, exposing your heart to repeated insults and injuries.

How to Change

There's good news for people with Type A or Type D personality: by altering your way of thinking and feeling about the world, as well as changing negative behaviors, you can work toward becoming more of a Type B individual and reap the associated benefits for your heart. You can begin making some heart-healthy changes by developing better ways of dealing with frustration and anger and by learning new strategies to manage your time and curb your impatience.

Managing Your Anger

Anyone can get angry—that is easy . . . but to do this to the right person, to the right extent, at the right time, with the right motive, and in the right way, that is not for everyone, nor is it easy.

—Aristotle

Anger is not all bad—it's an emotion everyone experiences at one time or another. The problem is, you may experience it too quickly in reaction to too many different events and at higher levels than may be realistically warranted. You may overreact, tending to see relatively minor incidents as major transgressions or acts of incompetence. When you are chronically angry, your body's physical and hormonal responses are also in a frequent state of irritability. As mentioned earlier, the end results of this process can lead to damaged or blocked arteries, heart attacks, or other symptoms of heart disease.

Holding this chronic anger in and not finding an appropriate way to express it can also lead to negative health consequences. It's been associated with higher total cholesterol levels, higher LDL cholesterol levels, and decreased cardiac blood flow. Silent ischemia, high blood pressure, and greater jumps in blood pressure during physical or mental stress have also been related to holding anger in. Interestingly, a recent study suggests that the most harmful way for you to cope with anger is to always express it the same way (Engebretson and Stoney 1995). If you always tend to hold it in or always tend to let it out in an explosive or hostile fashion, then you may be at greater risk of heart disease. The best approach seems to lie in being flexible. Sometimes it's best to let your anger drop and not express it. At other times, it's best to assertively express angry feelings.

Hostility is somewhat of a difficult concept to understand. To help you with this, think of hostility as composed of the following three dimensions:

1. A tendency to be suspicious and mistrustful of others

2. Having frequent angry feelings

3. Outward displays of aggressive actions

These dimensions may be expressed differently in you, depending on whether you are male or female. Most of the research on anger has involved men. But some recent studies suggest interesting findings for women. In general, women appear to get angry as often as men do and for similar reasons. However, they tend to express anger differently than men. While men are more likely to show anger with aggressive actions (like yelling, pounding their fists, throwing things), women are more likely to release the tension of anger with tears. Women more often keep their feelings to themselves or confide in a friend. Women also tend to feel more uncomfortable or guilty about angry outbursts than men do. Men more often believe that their hostility is justified and appropriate.

Not only is a hostile approach to life bad for your heart, but it also usually has negative consequences for your relationships. Chronic anger may drive away family members or friends. This then leaves you isolated and without the sources of social support that are so important for both your emotional and physical well-being.

There have been many books written on anger and ways to appropriately handle it. Several of these are listed in the Further Reading section at the end of the book. David Sobel and Robert Ornstein provide straightforward, practical suggestions for managing anger and hostility in healthy ways in *The Healthy Mind, Healthy Body Handbook* (1996). Some of their suggestions are included in the following discussion.

You may believe that anger is a response to a situation that has happened to you. Actually, anger is more accurately defined as an emotional response to your *perception* of what happened to you, or to your thoughts about it. How you view a situation determines whether you will feel angry or not. For example, if your thoughts about an interaction include this: "He probably did that on purpose—just to make me angry," then your emotional reaction will probably be anger. On the other hand, if your thoughts are something like these: "Well, maybe he did that thoughtlessly without meaning to," or "Maybe she is preoccupied with other concerns and that made her react that way," then you will be more able to avoid feeling angry. You will also be better able to communicate with other people without causing undue tension.

Drs. Sobel and Ornstein suggest that the next time you get angry, ask yourself the following questions:

- **Is this issue important enough for me to get angry about?** Consider whether this issue is an isolated incident or one that may tend to recur. Is it worth spending time and energy on? What's the worst that can happen as a result of the situation?

- **Does the available evidence support my anger?** In this regard, assess whether your response and expectations are realistic. Consider whether you may be confusing current feelings with something that happened in the past.

- **Will getting angry make a difference?** If it will, then you may want to assertively address your feelings. If it won't, then weigh the pros and cons of expressing your feelings. Though people often report feeling better just by venting feelings, sometimes getting angry and losing your cool is not useful for you at all. It may just increase your angry feelings and strain your heart and body, as well as your relationships.

Here are some additional techniques for controlling your anger:

- **Be assertive in expressing yourself.** Present your thoughts and feelings directly, using "I" statements rather than the more accusatory "You" statements.

- **Learn techniques for relaxation to decrease the tension associated with anger.** Use your favorite methods to relax, such as imagining a peaceful scene, taking a warm bath, or meditating. Try deep-breathing exercises or progressive muscle relaxation. These techniques are described in chapter 15.

- **Start exercising.** Exercise is one of the best ways to release the physical tension that accompanies angry feelings. Exercising may also release *endorphins*, the chemicals in the brain that are natural pain reducers and produce good, peaceful feelings. Drs. Sobel and Ornstein report that exercise may be especially beneficial for people who are hot reactors. A tendency for the cardiovascular system to react excessively to stress may be counteracted by the benefits of exercise.

- **Keep your sense of humor.** Sometimes laughter is the best medicine for undoing angry, tense feelings. The act of smiling or laughing in itself can lead to positive physical changes and produce pleasant feelings, even if you weren't happy to begin with. Try using exaggeration to help keep your perspective. When bothered by minor irritations, exaggerate your situation to extremes. This may help you laugh off minor annoyances. Watch out for unhealthy humor, such as sarcasm, cynicism, or contempt. Expressing humor in this way may actually intensify hostile or resentful feelings and will possibly hurt relationships.

- **Stay focused on the present.** During arguments, many people tend to begin with one issue but proceed to dredge up past mistakes, which only intensifies angry feelings. Limit your focus to the present issue and avoid making generalizations, such as "always" or "never."

- **Schedule a specific time as your "angry, worry time."** If you find yourself preoccupied with angry thoughts, set a specific time of about fifteen or twenty minutes during which you force yourself to think about the issues contributing to your anger. When angry thoughts come up at other times, set them aside and tell yourself you will think about them later. This technique gives you a greater sense of control over your feelings and is helpful in avoiding feeling overwhelmed by anger.

- **Keep a journal.** Writing down your feelings about your life, especially the distressing aspects, can allow you to more fully understand, process, and let go of angry feelings. Studies have shown that writing about distressing feelings may even boost your immune system (Whitehouse et al. 1996).

- **Learn how to forgive.** This does not mean that you will necessarily forget or excuse hurtful experiences. Instead, it means giving up resentments so they do not cast a shadow on your life and lead to enduring negative feelings.

If you've tried these or other strategies to deal with anger but are still plagued by irritability, agitation, or frequent hostile attitudes, then ask your doctor for a referral for counseling. Though you may have had an angry, hostile approach to life for many years, with practice, patience, and motivation you can learn healthier alternatives that lead to a more peaceful existence.

Managing Time Pressure

There are only twenty-four hours in a day, seven days in a week, fifty-two weeks in a year, and so on. You get the picture. Nevertheless, you may try to accomplish more tasks than are possible within a twenty-four-hour time period. Much of this problem comes from the many roles you play in your life and the many requirements and tasks that are put upon you—or that you take on yourself. Some people feel like they have no time at all. Others manage to get their work done and still have time left over for relaxing, pleasurable activities.

Poor time management can lead to ineffective decision-making, fatigue, and a feeling of being overwhelmed by the smallest details or demands. Listlessness or exhaustion can then result, which may affect your productivity in general. For example, you may miss deadlines at work because you spent many unproductive hours "spinning your wheels" and not getting far.

To reduce the immediate and long-term stress associated with time pressure, it's important to learn better time management strategies. The first step in eliminating time pressure is to analyze just how your time is spent. Use the chart on the following page to identify your activities in the course of a day. Accurately account for as much time in the day as you can, including travel, daydreaming, socializing, eating, grooming, and so on. Make several copies of the chart if your activities are significantly different on different days of the week.

When you actually identify and account for your time throughout the course of a day, you may be surprised at the amount of time you spend on various activities or by how inefficient your use of time is in certain areas. When you examine your time chart, does anything surprise you? Do you feel you have a balance between the amount of time spent in work versus the time spent in pleasurable, relaxing, and social endeavors? If not, is this achievable?

Make a list of your priorities and compare it to a list of activities that you spend a majority of your time on. Do the lists match up? For many people, they don't even come close. It's common for people to spend the majority of their time on work and other chores or duties of daily life and neglect those things they claim to value most. The end result of this may be a lack of closeness in personal relationships, stress due to lack of the positive experiences that would offset the challenges, and perhaps poor health. As the old saying goes, very few people look back on their life from their deathbed and wish that they had spent more time at work.

If you have experienced a heart attack or other form of heart disease, this is a wonderful time for you to learn to appreciate your life. Be glad you have it and take this as an opportunity to be sure you are making the most out of your life. The following strategies can help:

- **Prioritize the things you value most.** Spend less time in unimportant activities. Stay focused on what really matters to you in your life.

- **Organize yourself and your time.** Make lists of realistic goals; be liberal in crossing off any tasks you can do without. Use a calendar to schedule and plan activities and to help prevent you from agreeing to do too much.

- **Strive to achieve balance in your life** between challenging, draining responsibilities and pleasurable activities. On your calendar, schedule in regular relaxation time for yourself and time to build intimacy with significant others. Do not cancel this time. Reschedule if you can't keep the appointment.

Activities at Work   **Time Spent**

_____   _____

_____   _____

_____   _____

_____   _____

_____   _____

Activities at Home   **Time Spent**

_____   _____

_____   _____

_____   _____

_____   _____

_____   _____

Activities for Self   **Time Spent**

_____   _____

_____   _____

_____   _____

_____   _____

_____   _____

Travel   **Time Spent**

_____   _____

_____   _____

_____   _____

_____   _____

_____   _____

- **Be wary of perfectionism and spreading yourself too thin.** Instead of trying to get more out of life by doing more and engaging in as many activities as possible, get more out of life by slowing your pace down. Take time to "smell the flowers," whatever that may entail for you. Experiment with things like yoga, meditation, or spiritual involvement. Give up on unrealistic expectations that you can be the best for everyone all the time in every situation. Remember that the brightest stars tend to burn out the fastest, while the stars twinkling less fiercely provide steady illumination and warmth.

- **Learn to say no.** Ask for help when you need it and delegate as much as possible.

- **Live in the moment.** Don't dwell on past mistakes or events, and don't fret about the future either. Tune in to what is happening to you today and to who you are sharing today with. By doing this, you allow yourself the freedom to get the most out of your experiences without a constant feeling of rushing through each day.

- **Work on changing negative thought patterns.** If you notice that you are often making self-critical statements, such as "I'm absolutely worthless—I never get everything done that I should," replace these with encouraging reassurances like "No one is perfect, and just because I can't be perfect doesn't make me a bad person," or, "I'm doing the best I can, and I'm proud of that."

- **Procrastinate only when appropriate.** Sometimes it's fine to put things off. And, yes, it's even good to eliminate many tasks that are not necessary or important to you. On the other hand, it's not good to procrastinate on important tasks. In the end, you place even greater pressure on yourself. You'll probably find that many activities aren't as difficult or as unpleasant as you thought they would be. And once you get going, it's easier to continue.

Negative emotions such as anxiety and depression and the problematic personality styles discussed in this chapter can be highly damaging to your heart. The good news is that these difficulties can be altered and overcome. Read on to learn more about effectively managing the stress in your life.

15

Managing Stress

What Is Stress?

The word *stress* has become a fixture in our language. We make statements such as "I'm so *stressed* out" or "That was so *stressful*" as a commentary on the pressures we feel in our everyday lives. Stress is usually perceived as a negative occurrence, and the word is used interchangeably with tension or anxiety. But actually, *stress* refers to the demands, both positive and negative, that the environment places on you. Your body then responds in a complex manner to meet those demands. First, the sympathetic nervous system is activated. You may feel a surge or rush of adrenaline, a powerful hormone, and feel ready to "do battle." This causes your blood pressure to increase and your heart to beat faster. Your breathing becomes more rapid and your insulin level rises. The muscles in your stomach and intestines contract, which gives you those telltale "butterflies" or "that feeling in the pit of your stomach." These changes allow more oxygen and nutrients to be delivered to your muscles. This response is known as the *fight-or-flight* response and it is what helped humans in prehistoric times when they literally had to fight or flee in order to survive. When the acute event that triggered this response is over, the body's relaxation response is activated, resulting in a decrease in muscle tension, heart rate, breathing, and so on.

The same fight-or-flight response is triggered by everyday stressors. These stressors can be negative, like experiencing a death of a loved one, or positive, such as having a baby. Any change in your environment can activate the stress response so that you are better able to cope with the demands that are being placed on you. Even minor occurrences in your daily life, like getting stuck in traffic, can trigger the stress response. However, if your stress response is constantly activated, with little relief or return to a more relaxed state, your body can be harmed. Your body cannot withstand the pressure of being "on alert" all the time without wearing you down and increasing your chances of developing disease. You may experience signals that your body is experiencing too much stress.

Which of the following symptoms of stress have you experienced?

_____ Headaches	_____ Trouble concentrating
_____ Trouble sleeping	_____ Upset stomach
_____ Anxiety and worrying	_____ Digestion problems
_____ Appetite changes	_____ Mood swings
_____ Heart palpitations	_____ Losing temper often
_____ Crying more than usual	_____ High blood pressure
_____ Fatigue	_____ Tense muscles
_____ Feeling withdrawn from others	_____ Low motivation
_____ Feeling empty	_____ Nightmares
_____ Using more drugs or alcohol	

Some of these symptoms can be caused by medical problems. If you are experiencing any of the physical symptoms, in particular, it's important to be checked out by your physician. If there is no acute medical cause, then the symptoms may be related to your stress level.

One of the parts of your body that is reactive to chronic stress is your heart. Recall that when you are under stress, your heart beats faster and your blood pressure increases. The adrenaline surge causes blood pressure to rise, and without release of that tension through physical activity, the blood pressure drops off slowly until the next aggravation or stressor occurs. When this occurs too often over time, the body gives up and the blood pressure stays at a higher level. Over the long run, this clearly places strain on the heart. Chronic stress also causes your blood to clot more quickly. Recall that if blood clots quickly, it will be difficult for blood to flow smoothly through an artery that is blocked or partially blocked from fatty deposits (atherosclerosis). Many people with heart disease have a tendency to be *overreactive* to stress, which means they respond to even minor stressors with an automatic activation of their fight-or-flight response. For example, they might get agitated or tense about having to wait in line at the bank. It is like have your motor stuck in high gear even when some situations may only require first or second gear. As a result, you end up burning up a lot of unnecessary energy without effectively coping with the stressor. Your body ultimately pays the price for this extended high level of tension.

Techniques to manage stress can be divided into three categories: managing your physical reactions to stressful events, altering your thoughts and interpretations of events or stressors, and changing your behaviors related to the events. Each of these areas influence the other. For example, changes in your thoughts and interpretations can improve physical symptoms of tension. Similarly, better management of your physical tension can influence your behavioral reactions.

Managing Your Physical Reactions to Stress

It is almost impossible to change the statements you make to yourself or your behavior when you are in a high state of physical arousal. Therefore, the first step in dealing with stress is to control your physical arousal. Once you reduce the physical tension, you'll notice that you can concentrate better, have more energy, and feel more motivated to make other changes. Two good methods for managing physical tension are exercise and relaxation training. Refer to chapter 9 for more information on how exercise can reduce your physical tension. **Remember that you must consult with your physician before beginning any type of exercise program.**

Relaxation Training

The relaxation response is the opposite of the fight-or-flight response. This response quiets your body—your heart rate and breathing decrease, blood pressure drops, and muscles become relaxed. You can see, then, how this would benefit your heart.

Relaxation is also beneficial in managing your stress reactions, especially to minor events like getting stuck in traffic or waiting in line. Recall that many heart patients have a tendency to get their heart rate and blood pressure up when stressed. As you become more stressed and wound up, you are more likely to engage in behaviors that are also harmful to your heart such as smoking, or eating unhealthy foods. Many researchers, including Herbert Benson (1974), have shown that regularly using relaxation, in any form that calms your body, is beneficial to your heart.

Relaxation training helps people improve their ability to focus their attention on their bodies. Relaxation methods will enable you to effectively reduce both your mental stress and its physical signs. As you become more relaxed, you may be able to listen better to important things you want to say to yourself. Relaxation training is a self-control technique—you are in control of your stress.

Diaphragmatic Breathing

This technique involves breathing from your diaphragm instead of your chest. Your diaphragm is a muscle that is located just below your ribs. Breathing from the diaphragm involves slow, deep breaths where the diaphragm actually pulls and pushes air in and out of the lungs. Unlike the shallow, rapid, and tense breathing that occurs in the chest when you are anxious, breathing from the diaphragm promotes relaxation in the body.

There are many physical benefits to diaphragmatic breathing. First, this type of breathing makes relaxation on a physical level much easier to achieve. Second, this type of breathing is physically more efficient and subsequently increases the oxygen supply to the heart, brain, and other organs. And, third, by using this type of breathing, you make the process of healing your heart smoother and more complete. Here's how to do it:

1. Place your hand on your abdomen below your rib cage. This is where your diaphragm is located.

2. Take in a deep breath through your nose, hesitate for a moment, and then slowly exhale through your mouth. You should be able to feel your stomach moving out when you inhale and in when you exhale.

3. Repeat several deep breaths.

4. Remember to *slowly* but deeply inhale and slowly but *evenly* exhale. Avoid rapid, quick breaths. This can lead to hyperventilation.

5. You may wish to combine some imagery or a positive self-statement with the breathing exercise. For example, when you exhale, imagine letting all of the tension in your body go with the breath. You may imagine that when you inhale you are better able to take air in more fully.

The following is a relaxation exercise that combines diaphragmatic breathing with focusing on other parts of your body.

1. Find a comfortable chair in a quiet room.

2. Concentrate on your breathing, taking slow, deep breaths. Breathe through your nose, inhale, hold it, exhale slowly. Focus on your belly as it expands like a balloon when you inhale and deflates when you exhale.

3. Repeat this breathing for several minutes. Aim for a slow, comfortable rhythm.

4. As you concentrate on slowing down your breathing, also slow down your thinking and let your body sink into your comfortable chair.

5. Notice how relaxed your arms feel against the chair. Notice how your legs, back, and neck feel. Notice that your breathing is slow, deep, and regular.

6. You may imagine that you are inhaling fresh, clean air into your lungs, which are now able to expand more fully. Imagine each breath as a cleansing breath that is helping your body to heal itself.

7. As you exhale, imagine that you are releasing all the tension in your body. You are becoming more relaxed. Notice how the clean air can more fully enter your body and how your arms, legs, neck, and back begin to feel more relaxed. The tension slowly begins to fade each time that you exhale. Your body is cleansing and healing itself.

Progressive Muscle Relaxation

Progressive muscle relaxation was developed by Dr. Edmund Jacobson (1974). He found that you could achieve relaxation in your muscles by first tensing them. When you are working on tensing a particular muscle group, you need to try and keep all other muscle groups relaxed. Here's how it works:

1. Begin by lying down in a quiet and comfortable position.

2. Take several deep, cleansing breaths from the diaphragm.

3. Keep in mind that when you tense a muscle group you need to do so in an intense manner and should hold it for seven to ten seconds. You will then release the tension from the muscle group in an abrupt way. Enjoy the relaxed sensation for fifteen to twenty seconds.

4. Make two tight fists. Hold them (seven to ten seconds) and then release them (fifteen to twenty seconds).

5. Tense the muscles around your eyes by tightly holding your eyelids closed. Hold and release.

6. Open your mouth as widely as you can. Hold and release.

7. Raise your eyebrows as high as you can, tensing your forehead. Hold and release.

8. Tense your biceps by flexing the muscles. Hold and release.

9. Stiffen your arms, extend them to your side, and tense your triceps. Hold and release.

10. Shrug your shoulders by raising them up to your ears. Hold and release.

11. Pull your shoulder blades back as if you were sticking out your chest. Hold and release.

12. Tighten your stomach muscles. Hold and release.

13. Arch your lower back. Hold and release.

14. Squeeze the muscles of your buttocks together. Hold and release.

15. Flex your toes up toward you and tighten your calf muscles in your legs. Hold and release.

16. Curl your toes down towards the floor. Hold and release.

You will need to practice this exercise in a quiet, relaxed atmosphere before you can learn to do it in stressful situations. Initially, the exercise may take you twenty to thirty minutes to complete. With practice, however, you'll be able to reduce the time and achieve relaxation even in less than ideal situations.

Deep Breathing and Visualization

Your imagination and ability to daydream are powerful tools for reducing your stress. If you like, you can combine the dia- phragmatic breathing exercise with visualization for deeper overall relaxation. You may want to remember a version of the following visualization, or record yourself reading it out loud so that you can relax with your eyes closed. You might simply choose to create a scene of your own, once you get the idea. Remember to keep the details vivid.

You are walking on the beach. Feel the cool breeze that is blowing off the water. As you walk slowly along the shore, you can feel occasional droplets of water that spray up at you as the wind passes over the water. Feel the warmth of the sand between your toes. It feels coarse but smooth and gives way to your feet. You feel the tensing and relaxing of the muscles in your legs as you walk along. The sun is warm and soothing on your skin. You feel safe and relaxed. Now and then a bird calls out overhead, and you look up to see it soaring skyward. The scent of the water gently fills your nose and gives you a fresh, cleansing feeling.

As you look out over the water, you can see the sooth- ing rhythm of the water, gently lapping back and forth. The waves are rolling with a smooth, unhurried motion. You feel the beating of your heart with the same steady, slow rhythm of the waves, strong and sturdy and comfortable. You watch the free-flowing motion of the water and begin to imagine the same steady, free-flowing movement of blood in your arteries. No barriers or blockages. Nothing prevent- ing it from flowing comfortably and in an unhurried man- ner. You take in a deep breath of the fresh air, filling your lungs. Your chest expands without pain or tension. As you exhale, you can feel the tension being released from your body.

As you sit down on the beach, feel the warmth of the sand on your body. You feel strong and refreshed. You see your heart beating regular and strong, giving you the strength to handle life's stressors. You feel confident and proud of the control that you have over your body. You feel the improvements you have made on your body. Your stress level is lower. Your healthy diet has prevented your arteries from becoming clogged. You control the steady, free flow of blood through your arteries.

You remind yourself of all your strengths. You focus your thoughts on the positive things in your life. You feel the strength of those who support and love you. Pay attention to how strong you feel with the support of others, as if, at times, they're lifting and carrying you along like the waves. Remind yourself that you have control over your heart. You can keep it strong and safe. The clouds of pessimism and hopelessness are blown away by the steady wind. The only thing that remains, constant and steady like the sun, is your optimistic attitude. Like the sun, this optimism reflects off the water, touching all that surrounds you, and then returns back to you.

Pause for a few moments while you reflect on the steady and strong beating of your heart and the gentle, comfortable, and easy flow of the blood through your clean arteries. This blood carries energy, warmth, and strength to your mind. You are now more confident, content, productive, and happy as this rich blood bathes your mind with healthy substances.

Notice how much more relaxed and comfortable you have become and how much you have enjoyed being in this place. Focus on how relaxed your arms, legs, back, and neck feel. In a few moments you are going to bring yourself back by slowing down your breathing. Know that whenever you want to, you can bring yourself back to this spot.

Now begin slowing down your breathing while retracing your steps down the beach. When you are ready, count backwards from five to one. When you reach one, you will open your eyes, feeling relaxed, refreshed, alert, and ready to do whatever you want to do.

Begin practicing this visualization exercise twice a week for thirty minutes. If the example used here of walking on the beach is not particularly relaxing to you, then substitute some other place where you feel particularly relaxed and peaceful. The key to effective visualization is to make the imagery as vivid and real as you can. Therefore, when you are imagining this scene, or a scene of your own, it's important to try to imagine as many sights, smells, feelings, and sounds as you can. Try to place yourself into the scene in such a way that you can feel the breeze or sun, and hear the waves, the birds, and so on.

Try practicing your favorite exercises on a regular basis so that you become good at relaxing deeply and quickly. As with any skill, with time and practice you will improve.

Controlling Your Interpretations of Stressful Events

If you're like most people, you talk to yourself all the time. If this self-talk is accurate and realistic, you cope and function well. However, if your interpretation of a situation is false or exaggerated, you can feel stressed beyond what is healthy for the situation. It's important to begin evaluating your thoughts and interpretations by identifying what causes you to feel stressed.

Distinguish between the Stressors and Your Reactions

Many situations and events in life can cause you to react with a stress response. Some situations may be major stressors, while others are minor annoyances. Although these stressors can be divided into major and minor events, it is your interpretation and belief about these events that actually determines the level of stress you experience. For example, if you interpret a minor annoyance, like waiting in line, as a huge waste of time that you could be using more productively and spend the time in line looking at your watch and thinking about other places you need to be, then your stress level will probably rise. However, if you are able to interpret your waiting in line as a necessary experience and you use that time to focus your energy and thoughts on something positive, then your stress level is likely to stay low.

In an effort to better manage stress, it is important to separate stressors into major and minor events and then match your reaction and coping response to the type of stressor. Identify major stress events that you have been confronted with from the following list:

_____ Death of a loved one   _____ Buying a home

_____ Divorce   _____ Selling a home

_____ Illness of self   _____ Financial problems

_____ Illness of family member   _____ Legal problems

_____ Recent marriage   _____ Demanding job

_____ Birth of a new baby   _____ Victim of abuse

_____ Starting a new job   _____ Moving

_____ Losing a job   _____ Being a single parent

Identify which of the following minor irritants or daily stressors you react to:

_____ Dealing with traffic jams

_____ Being cut off by other cars in traffic

_____ Drivers not using signals, riding in wrong lanes, etc.

_____ Drivers not merging appropriately

_____ Waiting in lines

_____ Being behind someone in the supermarket express lane with more than twelve items

_____ Meeting work deadlines

_____ Being put on hold on the phone

_____ Dealing with solicitation phone calls

_____ Conflict with neighbors

What do you notice about yourself? Do you sweat the small stuff? Although you don't have complete control over the major and minor stressors in your life, you *do* have control over your reaction to them. Individuals with cardiac disease tend to overreact to even the minor annoyances of life. This overreaction puts you at a greater risk for future cardiac problems. Managing the stress caused by major life events can be challenging enough; then when you add an over-reactive response to minor events you can see how your body rarely gets a chance to idle in low gear.

In order to examine this overreactive style more closely, consider the following two scenarios and the different coping response by each individual:

Tom begins every day the same way. He jumps in his car and begins to rush to work. He rushes even if he is on schedule. He becomes quite annoyed when others drive too slow in the fast lane. He frequently weaves in and out of traffic because he feels agitated when he is held up by drivers in front of him. He often makes obscene gestures and uses profanity while yelling at drivers. His self-talk goes something like this: "Other drivers are idiots. Obviously they have no place important to go." By the time Tom arrives at work, his blood pressure is elevated, his heart rate is high, and his body is in a high-tension mode. He has initiated the fight-or-flight response. This reaction will be perpetuated as he arrives at work in this state and is confronted with deadlines and demands from his boss.

Since Tom does this often, his body rarely gets an opportunity to relax. This high state of chronic arousal puts him at risk for cardiac disease. Can you relate to Tom's feelings and behaviors? Do you get really stressed out in similar situations? Are you aware of your thoughts and physical reactions during these situations?

Jane often finds herself stuck in traffic on her way to work As she sits in the car constantly looking at her watch, she begins to feel her muscles tensing. She feels the beginning of a headache. These physical symptoms are used as a trigger for her to begin to talk to herself in an effort to relax. She makes self-statements such as, "I have no control over this traffic jam and getting upset is not going to get me to work any quicker." Or, "I need to relax or I won't be able to concentrate and be productive when I do get to work." She then turns on some music and tries to distract herself while waiting for the traffic to move.

The difference between these two scenarios lies in the way in which each person evaluates and interprets the stressor. In the first scenario, Tom's appraisal of and reaction to the minor stress of dealing with a traffic annoyance was disproportionate to the stressor. He triggered the fight-or-flight reaction in his body as if he were confronted with a life-or-death situation or a major trauma, such as divorce or death of a loved one.

In the second scenario, Jane was able to prevent her body from experiencing the fight-or-flight reaction by first recognizing that she was physically responding with muscle tension. She then used this tension as a trigger to move into healthy and proportionate self-talk. She used music as a distraction technique and her thoughts as a way to more accurately evaluate how getting stressed would not change the stressor. She realized that getting upset and physically ill was not going to cause the traffic to move and in the big picture of her life it was not a major crisis or stressor. By using this adaptive strategy, Jane was able to conserve her energy and coping abilities for the major events that she would probably be confronted with at some point in her life.

Avoid All-or-Nothing Thinking

People who suffer from cardiac disease or who are at risk for heart problems engage in all-or-nothing thinking. This involves using language like *should, never, always, ought to, need to,* and *must.* These words set up a standard that says if an event or person doesn't live up to an expectation, then the person is terrible or the situation is uncontrollable. In reality, it isn't the event or person that is bad but the standard that is set. The standard is irrational because people and situations are never all good or all bad, therefore you set yourself up to feel stressed, angry, or disappointed when they fail to meet this standard.

Albert Ellis (1975), a well-known psychologist, developed a theory about how irrational thoughts interfere with healthy coping. The theory suggests that engaging in negative self-talk—for example, evaluating yourself and your situation in a negative manner—increases your stress level and negatively influences your behavior and feelings. If you evaluate a situation based on irrational thoughts, then it is your thoughts—not the event itself—that cause you to feel anxious, angry, or depressed. At the core of irrational thinking is the belief that things are being done *to you*. However, situations simply occur; it is how you perceive their meaning and purpose that leads to stress. Therefore, if you change your irrational thoughts to more realistic and rational ones, you'll be able to reduce your physical reactions to stress and reduce negative feelings. Some of these irrational thoughts include the following:

- *I must be totally competent and perfect in everything I do.* Absolute, black-and-white thinking about perfection inevitably sets you up to fail, as this standard is irrational. When you feel less than perfect you become overwhelmed, stressed, and incapable of attempting anything new.

- *I always mess things up.* This type of extreme thinking leads people to take one instance and generalize it to everything in their lives. If one bad thing happens, then everything in their lives is awful. For instance, a person who tends to "awfulize" situations may, after missing a plane, make the following statements to him- or herself: "Why does this always happen to me?"; "I have a black cloud hanging over my head"; or "I never do anything right." This kind of thinking leads to intense irritation, tension, and anxiety.

- *I need to be loved and respected by everybody.* Although it's nice, and maybe preferable, to be loved and respected, you don't absolutely *need* it. It is unrealistic to think that *everyone* should feel that way about you. You may be reading this and thinking, "How ridiculous for anyone to want love from everybody." However, honestly ask yourself how frequently you are distressed when you don't feel respected by others, even if, rationally, you know that there will be situations where you encounter somebody that doesn't respect you. If you hold the irrational belief that everybody should respect you, then when you are actually confronted with somebody who doesn't respect you, self-doubt and stress can result.

Steps for Changing Extreme Irrational Thinking

1. **Objectively evaluate situations.** Go back and look at the circumstances and events that occurred at the time you were upset. Write down the facts—not what your impressions or ideas were. This will help you look at the situation more objectively. For example, "I had an argument with my boss." Then write down the facts that led to the argument and exact dialog that was spoken.

2. **Write down your self-talk.** For each fact in the situation, write down what your assumptions, beliefs, and worries were. What were you thinking, feeling, and saying to yourself? For example, "He is out to get me." "He looks at me as if I were stupid." "He makes me feel worthless."

3. **Evaluate the evidence for your self-talk.** Look at your self-statements and ask yourself, "What evidence do I have for this thought?" Attempt to recognize that it's your self-talk that is causing you the distress and not merely the situation. For example, "My boss may have challenged me about an issue but only my self-talk made me feel worthless."

4. **Ask yourself what the worst thing is that could happen as a result of the situation.** Directly confronting your worst fear will further help you to identify what your internal dialog is really about. For example, "The worst thing that could happen is that I may have to accept the consequences of my failures or my own feelings of inadequacy."

5. **Substitute more realistic self-talk.** When you are more clearly able to recognize your negative self-talk, you'll be able to substitute a healthy and realistic statement. For example, when you objectively evaluate the conflict with your boss and the negative self-talk that you engaged in, you may be able to say to yourself, "Accepting and facing the criticism of my boss is more productive than being defensive and making excuses for my performance."

Gain Control Over Your Need for Control

Everyone likes to feel in control. However, when you believe that you need to control all situations and people, you set yourself up for feelings of helplessness, anger, and frustration when those expectations are not met. Are you someone who likes to control your environment and others around you? Would others describe you as controlling? It's often difficult for us to see when we are being controlling. Although you may view yourself as "organized, decisive, and in charge," others may see you as controlling. Answer the following questions true or false:

_____ I believe that if I don't do things myself they won't get done right.

_____ Others seem to be more passive and indecisive than I am.

_____ People should plan and organize situations before taking action.

_____ People should have a very strong work ethic.

_____ I would rather work on projects alone than with a group.

Once you are able to accept the fact that you have little control over your environment and other people, you are more likely to actually *feel* in control. This may sound strange—that by letting go of your control needs you actually gain control—but it's true.

Consider situations where you may have struggled to get people to act the way you believed they should. Maybe you expected co-workers to put in the same amount of voluntary overtime as you do and you tried many ways to convince or encourage them to do so. Maybe you even ended up resenting them and spent energy in putting them down for "their lack of commitment." Perhaps you even carried this feeling of resentment home with you. You may have falsely believed that you should have had some control over the work ethic of others.

The reality is that you only have control over your own reactions to others and situations. By changing your thoughts and interpretations and managing your physical reactions to situations, you gain control over yourself. Feeling helpless, frustrated, and stressed will fade as you begin to feel more in control. The goal is to let go of trying to control things that are beyond your control in an attempt to gain control of yourself.

Changing Your Stressful Behaviors

The way you communicate with others can contribute to stress in your life. If you feel that others aren't listening to you or that your needs aren't being recognized, you may react in a way that actually increases your stress level. For example, frequently when people feel that others are not listening to them, they respond by nagging or arguing their position with more intensity. This response usually only serves to escalate conflict or tension. Learning better techniques to communicate, using assertiveness skills to stick up for your rights, and using effective problem-solving techniques can all reduce stressful interactions.

Communication Skills

You may experience stress during interactions with others because you do not feel equipped with the skills to effectively communicate. Doubting your skills and your ability to handle yourself during interpersonal interactions only serves to make you feel more self-conscious, which then feeds into feelings of stress. Here are five important skills that may help you feel more at ease when interacting with others.

Reading Nonverbal Cues

Part of the discomfort that people experience in social situations is often a result of their misinterpretation of others' body language. Have you ever said to yourself, "They look bored when I am talking" or "They seem like they are evaluating me"? These statements can stem from overinterpretations or misperceptions of body language. For example, your co-worker may be yawning or not making great eye contact with you because she is lacking sleep or because she is uncomfortable in social situations and not because she finds you boring. It's important to not base all of your interpretations on body language alone. It's also important that you pay attention to your own body language. Perhaps you are not aware of the signals that you are sending to others. For example, you may be physically separating yourself from others based on where you stand. Or perhaps you tend to make poor eye contact with others or you cross your arms in front of you as a way to keep separate from others. If you are doing these things, you may be feeding into your own sense of isolation, discomfort, and perceptions of being negatively evaluated by others. Reading other people's nonverbal cues and recognizing your own are two parts of the same skill—and that skill takes practice to develop.

Get together with a friend or a family member whom you trust. Ask the other person to observe your nonverbal cues and then ask for feedback on what he or she observes. Likewise, reverse roles and provide the other person with feedback on what you observe.

What did the other person tell you about your nonverbal cues?

_____

_____

What did you observe about the other person's nonverbal cues?

_____

_____

_____

Active Listening Skills

Good listening skills will help you interact more completely with others, which will in turn make you feel more comfortable in social situations. Although most people believe that they are good listeners, they usually are not. Listening is a skill that, like any other skill, requires *practice.* Being a good listener means more than just hearing what the other person is saying, it means fully understanding the content of what the other person is saying in a nonjudgmental way. Use the following hints to improve your listening skills:

- Avoid being judgmental and evaluative when listening to others.

- Avoid planning your next response while the other person is still talking. If you're thinking about how to respond, you're probably not listening very well.

- Avoid assuming that you know what the other person is saying. Once you start assuming you understand, you stop listening to the content.

- Repeat back, in your own words, what you think the other person has said. Don't repeat verbatim like a parrot, but rather summarize the essence of what you heard. Convey your understanding of what has been said. For example,

  Joe: My boss gave me another assignment to complete while Stan appears to have time on his hands.

  Carole: You seem irritated at what appears to be unequal work assignments.

  Joe: I'm not just irritated, I'm angry at the unequal treatment.

In order to repeat what you've heard, you need to pay close attention to what is being said to you. In other words, you need to engage in active listening. Moreover, by repeating back to the other person the essence of what you've heard, you provide the opportunity to clarify any misunderstandings. In the example, Carole correctly identified Joe's dissatisfaction about the unequal work assignments. However, she thought he was merely irritated by the situation but in reality he was angry. By repeating back to Joe what she understood, Carole gave him the chance to more fully explain his position. This helped her more accurately and fully understand what was being conveyed to her.

Initiating and Maintaining a Conversation

It may be difficult for you to go up to someone and just start a conversation. You may feel awkward and unsure of where to begin. An easy rule to follow is to start conversations with open-ended questions. These are questions that can't be answered with a simple yes or no. If you ask closed questions, or questions that can be answered with a yes or no response, you might end the discussion. That is, after the other person has responded, the dialogue is limited. Open-ended questions ask *what, when, where,* and *how.* Avoid overusing *why* questions, as this can put people on the spot or make them feel defensive. Following are examples of a conversation using closed and open-ended questions.

Closed Question

Jack: Do you like red wine?

Sue: Yes.

Open-Ended Questions

Jack: What kind of wine do you like?

Sue: I usually like red wine but on certain occasions I drink white.

Jack: They serve an excellent white wine here.

Sue: How do you know so much about wine?

Jack: I took a wine-tasting class.

You can see from this example that conversation flowed much smoother and with greater ease when open-ended questions were being used. They provided the opportunity for there to be more dialogue and interaction between the two people.

Assertiveness Skills

Asserting your needs, feelings, and opinions will help you keep your stress level down. If you believe that others' opinions and views are better or more interesting than yours, then you will behave accordingly. Being assertive will help you feel more confident, and this will be reflected in the way you handle yourself in social situations. As a result, you will feel more relaxed. Use the following strategies and suggestions to improve your assertiveness skills.

- **Keep in mind that assertiveness is not aggressiveness.** Assertiveness is a balance between the two extremes of aggressiveness and submissiveness. People who act in an aggressive style demand and expect others to do exactly what they want. Those who act in a submissive style give up their own beliefs, opinions, and wants to those of others. They feel guilty asking for what they want, as if others' needs are more important than their own. Assertive people respect others' views and feelings but also value and respect their own.

- **Look others directly in the eyes when talking to them and maintain an open posture.** This will be easier to do if you reinforce for yourself that what you are saying is important. Don't behave as though you don't value what you're saying. But, also, don't assume a posture that says you are absolutely right. For example, this might include glaring at others when speaking or ending your statement as if there is no questioning or doubting your words.

- **Be specific when making requests.** Vague requests or comments can often be misinterpreted by others or simply ignored. If your request is specific and direct, there will be little room for confusion. For example, instead of asking for someone's help in general, specifically state with *what* you want help, *when*, and for *how* long.

- **When discussing an opinion or making a request, use statements that begin with I.** When you use "I" statements, it is more likely that others will be receptive to hearing what you have to say. For example, *I feel...*, *I want...*, or *I think...*, and so on. Statements that start out with "you," such as, *You said ...* or *You think ...* tend to put other people on the defensive and less likely to be open to what you are saying.

- **Observe the behavior, nonverbal cues, and conversations of others who appear to be quite comfortable in social situations.** Examine how your nonverbal cues, behavior, and conversation are similar or different from their style.

List a few people you know who seem attentive and at ease when interacting with others.

_____

_____

Which of their characteristics gives you the impression that they are at ease with others and able to truly listen to others?

_____

_____

What similarities do you notice between your style in social situations and their style?

_____

_____

_____

What differences do you notice between their style and yours?

_____

_____

_____

Practice modeling the characteristics that you feel help them interact with others without becoming stressed. For example, if they seem to assume a certain body posture, practice that posture when you are alone and then when you are in a social situation.

Problem-Solving Skills

Another technique for managing stressors is use effective problem-solving techniques. Tackling a problem in a systematic manner will make it seem more manageable and less overwhelming.

1. **Recognize that there is a problem.** The first step in problem solving is to acknowledge that a problem exists and decide that you are not going to avoid dealing with it.

2. **Define the problem in as much detail as possible.** Be specific and include how you feel about the situation.

3. **Brainstorm some solutions.** This means making a list of possible solutions *without* evaluating whether they are good or bad. The more ideas you can generate, the more likely it is that you'll find one that works. This is a good time to get ideas from other people as well.

4. **Evaluate each of the solutions.** Go back and rank your possible solutions in terms of what you think is plausible. Think about the positive and negative consequences of each option. There is no perfect solution, but there may be one or two that will work best for you.

5. **Try out one of the solutions and decide whether or not it worked.** You may have to try it out a few times before it works. Evaluate the situation to see what worked and make adjustments as needed. If it was not effective, go back to steps 3 and 4 and try another solution. Remember, there is no perfect solution, but one of your options should be fine.

Try out this procedure for a problem that you are currently experiencing or have experienced.

What is the problem?

_____

_____

Define your problem in detail. Include all aspects of it—when it happens, who is involved, how it affects you and others, and so on.

_____

_____

_____

_____

Brainstorm possible solutions.

_____

_____

_____

Evaluate these options by listing advantages and disadvantages.

_____

_____

_____

_____

Pick the most appropriate solution and identify whether it worked or not. List problems and what adjustments you need to make. (Go back to previous steps if it did not work.)

_____

_____

_____

Spirituality

"The man who has no inner life is a slave of his surroundings."
—Henri Frederic Amiel

We include a section on spirituality and finding meaning in life because we have been impressed with the people who've been successful in making difficult lifestyle changes while coping with a life-altering event like a heart attack. They, and their families, often come out of the crises with renewed vigor, purpose, and meaning in their lives. They do not spend an overly large amount of time being bitter about what happened to them nor do they stay stuck in an endless cycle of repeating the same lifestyle patterns they had before their heart attack. Rather, they go about systematically changing their lives without a lot of attention. Their commitment to change often seems to come from a strength within. This is from their spiritual side, no matter how they define spirituality. If you have a deep spiritual side to you, then this section will reinforce what you already know. If you do not believe in this concept, do not feel compelled to read this section. Actively managing your risk factors will be adequate in reducing your chances of having a heart attack.

The search for purpose or meaning in life has plagued people for centuries. The process of this quest can leave you feeling either exhilarated and renewed at the realization of meaning or empty at your inability to find this meaning or purpose. Think about some of the language that is used when we talk about meaning and purpose in our lives. We refer to "feeling something missing." While we may not be able to put a label on what is missing, we are aware of a feeling of incompleteness. If you have felt this way, it could come from not having a sense of purpose or meaning in your life. These feelings are also triggered when you suffer a life-altering crisis or a brush with death like a heart attack. You may find yourself asking questions such as, "Why did this happen to me?" "What am I going to do now?" and "What if I have another heart attack?"

Consider the following vignette:

David went to the first counseling session appearing to be somewhat anxious. When he told his story, he began with an apology. He stated that he was sorry that he'd made the appointment because he felt that he might actually be wasting his time and the therapist's. He reported that he didn't know if he really had a problem or a *real* reason for needing counseling. He went on to say that he is a successful attorney in a rather large firm. Professionally, he felt fulfilled by his work and believed that he had accomplished many of the career goals he had set for himself. He felt personally gratified by his work and received much support and recognition from his peers. In his personal life, he had been happily married for sixteen years and had three healthy children. He believed his life to be busy but balanced, as he made time with the family a priority and scheduled days off for special activities with the children. He and his wife took one weekend out of the month to get away and nurture their relationship. He had little financial worries and a large group of supportive friends. The year before, he had suffered his first heart attack. He had made many lifestyle changes including adding a regular exercise program into his life and adjusting his diet. His last doctor's visit went well and he was currently free of any physical symptoms. He went on to say, "So, why am I here? I'm not sure. Despite many of the positive and satisfying aspects in my life I feel anxious about my future and whether or not I'll have another heart attack. Something feels unfinished. I'm embarrassed to be here trying to explain a problem that I can't see or describe—except to say I don't feel an inner sense of happiness."

Does this feeling that something is not quite right or complete in your life sound familiar? Do you feel that your life has all the ingredients but is lacking in someone or something to guide you through the *process* of living? Like David, many feel an emptiness or that something is missing inside of them. This place inside is often described as the soul or the place where your spirit resides. The spirit is traditionally believed to be the vital force within that gives us vigor and energy and provides us with a sense of determination and courage. This spirit or energy can come from many different avenues: nature, organized religions, prayers to whomever it is that you believe in, or from meditation, which allows you to focus your energy and attention in the present. Each of these different sources of spiritualism shares a common goal of increasing your internal energy source, which allows you to live more fully in the present. By more fully experiencing the *process* of living, you'll end up feeling more complete, less stressed, and happier at a core level of your being. Spirituality can help you

- Achieve peace of mind
- Find some purpose or meaning in your life
- Find strength and support
- Help you feel more connected to others

You can develop your spirituality or strengthen it through the following ways:

- Regular attendance at your church, temple, mosque, or any other organized spiritually based activities
- Reading inspirational literature on a regular basis
- Prayer in whatever form on a regular basis
- Practicing meditation as often as possible

Meditation

The practice of meditation began several thousand years ago in India. It was originally a method of improving one's spiritual nature by connecting with a Higher Power, becoming more "enlightened," and achieving peace of mind. While it is still practiced as a form of spirituality, it is also helpful to use as a form of relaxation. Meditation focuses your attention on the present, the here and now, and allows you to let go of thinking about the past or future for a short period of time. If you find that your mind is always racing or that you are angry or worried about things over which you have no control, this technique can be helpful. Herbert Benson (1974), who has done much research on the effects of relaxation on the cardiac response, studied meditation as a form of relaxation and found that it decreased heart rate, blood pressure, breathing rate, oxygen use, and metabolic rate. This is particularly noteworthy for heart patients because anything that reduces the strain on your heart will benefit you in the long run.

How to Practice Meditation

1. Find a quiet place to sit where there is little noise from the outside. You may try playing a tape of soft music or nature sounds in the background.

2. Sit comfortably in a chair with your feet on the floor, hands resting on your thighs with your palms up and fingers relaxed. Do not sit too rigidly because this will strain your muscles. On the other hand, do not lie down because you may fall asleep.

3. Try to reduce any muscle tension you may feel by using progressive muscle relaxation or slowly rotating your head clockwise or counterclockwise a few times while breathing deeply.

4. Select some focus for your attention. This can be a word or phrase of your own choosing like "one," "peace," or "I am healthy," or you can simply focus on your own breathing or a mental image.

5. Concentrate on whatever you've chosen. If it is a word or your breathing, then close your eyes. Repeat your word each time that you exhale. If other thoughts or images pop into your mind, do not try too hard to block them out. Simply imagine that they are leaves floating in and out of your vision.

6. Expect your mind to be distracted; this is normal. The more you practice, the better you will be at redirecting your attention back to the simple word, your breathing, or image when your mind wanders.

7. When you first begin to practice meditation, plan on doing it for about five to ten minutes at a time and gradually work your way up to twenty minutes or more.

8. Don't worry about whether you're doing it right or not, or whether it is working. Just focus your attention on redirecting your thoughts gently back to repeating the word or focusing on the image.

Meditation is one of many techniques you can use to become more spiritual, calm your mind during periods of stress, and relax. Like the other forms of relaxation presented in this chapter, such as progressive muscle relaxation and visualization, it will take practice to learn how to meditate so that you can incorporate it into daily practice. But, for those who use meditation on a regular basis, they find it a helpful tool in feeling calm and at peace.

The Value of Humor

"Laughter is like inner jogging. Not only does it exercise our facial muscles, but it also releases tension. It reminds us to breathe deeply. When we laugh, anger fades and our perspective changes."
—Beth Wilson Aavedra

Humor can be one of the best stress relievers. Scientifically, laughter has been shown to release endorphins—the body's own natural pain-killer and feel-good chemical. From a physical standpoint, laughing is like an aerobic exercise. Researchers have shown that one hundred good belly laughs have the same health benefits as fifteen minutes on a stationary bicycle (Fry 1997). Laughter has also been shown to strengthen the immune system so it can fight off viral and bacterial infections. Good, solid laughter can even increase the natural killer cells of the body that destroy abnormal precancerous cells. Laughter really is good medicine.

From an emotional standpoint, using humor can be a good coping strategy. When you laugh about something, you can momentarily forget your tension, and your body automatically relaxes. Humor can also give you a fresh approach to life's daily stressors. It can help you keep a sense of proportion and perspective about situations in which you find yourself. After all, there will be many things—other people's actions or life events—that will be out of your control.

How do people actually develop a sense of humor? Learning to laugh begins during infancy. Physically, a baby is able to laugh at about three to six months of age. Laughter at this developmental stage begins with a physical response to being tickled and, with increased age, to visual puns, such as putting a hat over your face. The type of humor that children respond to progresses from basic knock-knock jokes to more sophisticated riddles and jokes. During adolescence, the type of jokes that elicits laughter usually involves putting others down or having someone being the butt of the joke.

Differences between males and females with regard to use of humor begin during adolescence and persist into adulthood. In 1990, Dr. Lefcourt found that when women used humor as a strategy for coping with stress, they had lower systolic blood pressure readings than women who did not use humor as a coping strategy. However, when looking at men he found that the opposite was true. Men who used humor to cope had higher systolic blood pressure readings than men who did not. Why is this so? Lefcourt speculated that when using humor, women tend to laugh more at themselves or at situations as a way of promoting social closeness and support. On the other hand, men tend to use humor that puts others down as a way of keeping a social hierarchy of control. This need for control and an attitude that reflects hostility are major risk factors for cardiovascular disease.

If you use humor when coping with your heart disease, this does not suggest that your condition is funny or that you are not taking it seriously. Instead, it is a healthy way of distancing yourself from difficult information about your pain and suffering. This distancing allows you to take a break from your current distress while at the same time mobilizing your resources for future coping needs. On an emotional level, humor can bring enjoyment to life and dramatically interfere with the thoughts and feelings of depression and anxiety related to your heart disease. In other words, it's difficult to feel depressed and anxious while you're laughing.

Find ways to laugh every day. Read funny cartoons and stories, listen to your favorite comedians, watch a situation comedy on television, or see a funny movie. Keep in mind, though, that not all humor is suited for everyone. Therefore, it's important to find the right type of humor for you. For example, shows such as the *Drew Carey Show*, *Seinfeld*, and *Frasier* are a great source of humor for those who like quick-witted and slightly off-color humor. Or old-fashioned slapstick, such as *Laurel and Hardy*, may be more up your alley. Much of what makes for good humor are those books, movies, or sitcoms that allow you to laugh at yourself or the social mistakes of others. This type of humor can give you social cues about appropriate behavior and can also teach you that it is acceptable to make mistakes at times. This attitude will lead you to be more tolerant of others and, ultimately, will be healthy for your heart. So go ahead and laugh.

PART 5

Coronary Heart Disease in Women

Heart disease is the single most common cause of death in both men and women. Until recently, the "and women" was not appreciated.

—Dr. Elizabeth Barrett-Connor

16

Women and Coronary Heart Disease

The American Heart Association has referred to heart disease in women as a "silent epidemic." Most people, and even many medical professionals, are not aware of how prevalent heart disease is in women. In fact, women tend to be much more afraid of dying from breast cancer, or another form of cancer, than of suffering a heart attack. When a woman feels a lump in her breast, her first fear is typically of cancer. However, if a woman feels pains in her chest, she is more likely to assume it's indigestion, a muscle strain, or "nerves" than to think it's a heart attack. What you are learning by reading this book, however, is that being female does not mean you are not at risk for heart disease. Consider the following commonly held myths, as well as the facts that dispute them:

Myth: Heart disease is primarily a man's disease.

Fact: Cardiovascular disease, of which coronary heart disease is one type, is the major cause of death for women in the United States. Considering all ages, it leads to more deaths in women than men each year and accounts for almost 50 percent of the total deaths in women aged fifty and older. Since 1984, the number of deaths from cardiovascular disease for women has continued to outpace those for men—the difference in deaths is currently estimated to be over thirty-five thousand per year. The belief that it is a man's disease is in part related to the fact that, for many years, studies done on heart disease have involved primarily men. Historically, only about 10 to 25 percent of persons included in studies of heart disease have been women. Because heart disease tends to occur in men about a decade earlier than it shows up in women, it has probably been viewed as more important or more prevalent in men. The first signs of heart disease generally make their appearance in men in their mid forties, while women are usually in their mid fifties or later when the first signs of heart disease appear. After women reach menopause, usually around age fifty, their rates of heart disease climb steeply and become roughly equal to that of men by age sixty-five to seventy.

Myth: Women are more likely to die of breast cancer, or another type of cancer, than of heart disease.

Fact: Women are about eleven times more likely to die of heart disease than breast cancer. Heart disease claims more lives of women in the United States each year than all forms of cancer combined.

Myth: The symptoms of a heart attack are the same for women and men.

Fact: There are established gender differences throughout the course of heart disease in how symptoms are presented.

If you are surprised by these facts, you're not alone. A 1995 Gallup poll for the National Center of Health Statistics (Price 1995) shows just how confused people's perceptions of heart disease are. It showed that four out of five women aged forty-five to seventy-five years—80 percent of those polled—did not know that heart disease is the main cause of women's deaths. Worse yet, about one-third of the physicians surveyed did not know this either. When women were asked to identify the most common causes of death in women in the United States, the majority responded by estimating that almost 50 percent of deaths are due to breast cancer, with about another 20 percent due to other forms of cancer. They believed that less than 5 percent of yearly deaths in women were due to heart disease. The actual statistics are vastly different! Contrary to women's beliefs, about 34 percent of deaths in women are due to heart disease, with only 4 percent due to breast cancer and about 17 percent due to other types of cancer such as lung, uterine, or ovarian. Over a lifetime, your overall risk of dying from heart disease is 23 percent; your lifetime risk of dying from breast cancer is about 4 percent.

Fortunately, researchers are coming around, and there is an ever growing focus on the topic of heart disease in women. This was prompted by the American Heart Association's educational campaign in 1989 on women and heart disease. Currently, there are several large, long-term projects underway exploring the risk factors for heart disease in women, as well as the best ways to diagnose and treat heart conditions in women.

What's Different for Women?

Many conclusions about heart disease have been drawn from studies that included primarily men. So it's important to remember that these results may or may not apply to women as well. Some recent studies have suggested that women may have different initial symptoms of heart disease than men. Also, there seem to be differences in risk factors, referral rates for various diagnostic tests and treatment, and recovery rates. Read on to learn more about what is known so far about these differences.

Warning Signs of Coronary Heart Disease

For men, the first sign of heart disease is often a crushing chest pain that has been likened to having an elephant sit on your chest. Observations of women over the years have suggested that they are less likely to report intense, crushing chest pain and more likely to have the following signs of heart disease or attack:

- Chest discomfort; a feeling of tightness in the chest or throat
- Feeling short of breath, with or without exertion; waking up breathless at night
- Nausea; symptoms of indigestion
- Decreased energy; fatigue on a regular basis

Symptoms of a heart attack in women may be more vague than those often occurring in men. As a woman, you may have more difficulties assessing your symptoms. Additionally, physicians may not recognize symptoms of heart disease in women as quickly as in men. For example, a recent poll (cited in Hales 1997) suggested that approximately one-third of primary care doctors incorrectly believe that there is no difference between symptoms of heart disease in men compared to those reported most often by women. The Framingham heart study, which has followed women for about twenty years, found that nearly one-third of women's heart attacks are not detected at the time they occur (Kannel 1986). In addition, women may be less likely than men to experience any warning signs prior to sudden episodes of cardiac arrest. Women who survived cardiac arrest were less likely to have underlying heart disease, or blocked arteries, than men. In over 60 percent of the cases, cardiac arrest was the first sign of heart disease—their hearts just stopped without warning (Albert et al. 1996).

Doctors need to be better educated about the differences in symptoms of heart disease between men and women. You can do your part by becoming familiar with these differences and by not minimizing or neglecting "vague" signs. When symptoms such as chest discomfort, pain in the throat, neck, or arm, or shortness of breath occur regularly or for more than a few minutes, seek medical help quickly.

Prognosis or Recovery Rates

In general, the prognosis, or health outcomes, for women after a heart attack are worse than for men. Consider the following:

- About 44 percent of heart attacks are fatal for women, compared to 31 percent for men. At older ages, women are about twice as likely to die within a few weeks of a heart attack (American Heart Association 1995).

- In the year after a heart attack, women have a 20 percent chance of having another heart attack, compared to a 16 percent chance for men.

- Women are more likely to be depressed, anxious, stressed, and unhappy with their social support after a heart attack than men. Women tend to be less satisfied with their lives after a heart attack, regardless of age or severity of the attack.

- For African-American women, the dangers are even greater: death rates for heart disease are 69 percent higher than for white women.

- Women are less likely than men to be referred to a cardiac re-habilitation program, and those women who do attend are more likely to drop out than men.

- Return-to-work rates after a heart attack are lower in women than in men.

These differences may be due in part to age differences. On the average, women tend to have heart attacks at age sixty-nine, compared to an average age in men of fifty-nine years.

Why Do Men Get Heart Disease Earlier than Women?

Men's risks for heart disease begin to bypass women's risks after adolescence and continue to be higher until about the mid forties. Between the ages of thirty-five and forty-five, men are about three to four times more likely to develop heart disease than women. Sometime around the mid forties to early fifties, women's risks for heart disease begin to climb more steeply than men's. Around age sixty-five to seventy, women and men have roughly the same odds of heart disease.

Why do women's risks climb? It's widely accepted that this is primarily due to physical changes associated with menopause. During the premenopausal years, estrogen appears to protect women from suffering the heart attacks men may experience in their forties and fifties. Estrogen is believed to prevent a buildup of plaque in the arteries by increasing levels of HDL cholesterol, and by decreasing levels of the more dangerous LDL cholesterol. Estrogen may also protect the heart in other ways, such as by relaxing and dilating blood vessels.

Once past menopause, however, women's levels of estrogen drop, and they hit a danger zone of their own. Postmenopausal women have been shown to have higher rates of heart disease than premenopausal women.

According to Dr. Jay Sullivan (Speroff et al. 1997) of the University of Tennessee, men may be at greater risk of heart disease earlier in their lives because of lifelong difficulties with cholesterol levels. The levels of the good, HDL cholesterol in young men appear to decline steeply as they go through puberty. From this point on, the blood vessels of men may be prematurely clogged with buildup of the LDL cholesterol. Hence, men have earlier atherosclerosis, or narrowing of the arteries, than women.

Men may also have a greater physical and cardiovascular reaction to stress than women. This is the notion of the hot reactor, described in chapter 14. Over long periods of time, this overreacting to stress can lead to heart disease earlier in men. Men may also engage in more health-harmful behaviors than women, putting themselves at risk for a variety of physical disorders.

Traditional Risk Factors

Factors such as high cholesterol, high blood pressure, smoking, obesity, and high stress levels increase risks for developing heart disease in both men and women. However, these factors may influence you differently based on whether you are female or male.

Smoking

Cigarette smoking appears to put women at greater risk of heart disease than men. Results from the large Framingham heart study suggest that a fifty-five-year-old female smoker is more likely to have a heart attack than a fifty-five-year-old male smoker. Women who smoke have an estimated 15 percent higher risk of heart attack than men who smoke. If you smoke, you are from two to six times more likely to have a heart attack than a nonsmoking woman, and your risk increases the more cigarettes you smoke per day.

Cigarette smoking appears to rob women of their hormonal protection against heart disease by increasing the rate at which estrogen is broken down in the body. If you are a woman smoker, then you may go through menopause one or two years earlier than if you were a nonsmoker. Smoking contributes to heart disease in women as early as in their twenties or thirties. If you use birth control pills (oral contraceptives), and you smoke, you are engaging in what may be a particularly lethal combination: studies estimate that you are up to **forty times** more likely to have a heart attack and **twenty-two times** more likely to have a stroke, especially if you are over age thirty-five.

Oral contraceptives alone increase risk of heart disease by leading to conditions like increased weight and blood pressure, and by reducing levels of the protective HDL cholesterol. They also may contribute to spontaneous blood clot formation in veins or arteries. Recall that without enough of the HDL cholesterol, fatty plaques can form on the walls of your arteries, thereby narrowing them. If a blood clot forms, then the flow of blood through that narrowed artery is restricted or blocked and the result is a heart attack. Risks of this happening are higher if you also smoke, have diabetes or high blood pressure, or if you are over age thirty-five.

Roughly twenty-three million women in the United States smoke cigarettes. Women are not stopping smoking as quickly as men, and more adolescent girls currently smoke than boys. If you are avoiding quitting smoking because of fears of gaining weight, keep this in mind: you would have to gain about fifty pounds to put the same strain on your heart that you do by smoking. So do yourself—and your heart—a favor, and quit smoking. Refer to chapter 10 for useful advice on how to quit.

Weight

Women are twice as likely as men to experience significant weight gain. More than one-third of white women and almost half of African-American women are overweight. One study found that 70 percent of heart disease in heavy women was due to excessive body fat (Baron-Faust 1995; Wenger, Speroff, and Packard 1993). If you are overweight and also smoke, you may be five times more likely to develop heart disease than a nonsmoker of the same weight.

High Blood Pressure

Women with high blood pressure (hypertension) are up to eight times more likely to have a heart attack or stroke. If you are African-American, Latina, or Native American, your risks associated with high blood pressure are even greater. High blood pressure occurs in about 10 percent of pregnant women. Very high blood pressure can occur along with rapid weight gain; swollen ankles; and protein found in the urine, which is known as *toxemia*, or *pre-eclampsia*, and can lead to stroke.

Cholesterol (HDL, LDL)

Levels of the "good" cholesterol, HDL, may be one of the strongest predictors of heart disease in women. For example, women with low levels of HDL and high levels of triglycerides tend to have high blood sugar and high blood pressure and are at increased risk of heart disease—even if total cholesterol levels are within the normal range.

Dr. S. Casscells (1996) at the University of Texas has recently begun using a new method of screening for heart disease in women. Using a blood test, levels of the following factors are measured. Dr. Casscells reports that each of these factors appears more associated with heart disease in women than in men:

- Cholesterol (HDL, LDL)

- Triglycerides

- Lipoprotein(a)—high levels of this lipid, or fat, are more predictive of heart disease in women than men.

- Fibrinogen—this factor is related to blood clotting. It has been shown to be a risk factor for heart attack and death from heart attack. High levels of this substance are more often found in women than in men. Levels can be decreased by reducing total calorie intake and by consuming olive oil.

- Homocysteine—high levels of this substance lead to fewer clot-preventing or clot-dissolving substances in the blood. High homocysteine levels are associated with heart attacks, strokes, and circulatory problems. This factor may be as powerfully related to heart disease as high blood pressure, smoking, or cholesterol. Folic acid, a B vitamin found in fruits and vegetable, appears to normalize high levels of homocysteine.

- Serum magnesium—low levels of magnesium in the blood are more common in women, especially after menopause or pregnancy. It can be taken in tablet form to correct deficiencies. Levels of magnesium in the blood influence blood pressure, stickiness of the blood, and levels of stress hormones in the blood. Deficiencies of magnesium can lead to narrowed coronary arteries, irregular heart rhythms, and risk of cardiac death.

Dr. Casscells believes that lack of identification of these factors in women may be one reason why the death rate due to heart disease is not falling as fast for women as it is for men. When the risks are identified, they can be modified by making changes in your lifestyle. You can reduce risks associated with these factors by reducing total fat and calories in your diet while increasing vegetables, fruits, and perhaps by taking vitamin supplements or medications. The dietary changes can increase levels of HDL cholesterol, while decreasing levels of triglycerides, lipoprotein(a), and LDLs. New research also suggests that vitamin E may be more effective for women than it is for men in reducing risks for a heart attack (Casscells 1996; Kushi et al. 1996).

Though women tend to have poorer outcomes after a heart attack than men, the good news for women is that their heart health may respond better to lifestyle changes. Dr. Dean Ornish has reported that women appear to have better chances of stopping or even reversing heart disease than men. This may be true even if women make fewer changes in diet, exercise patterns, and stress management than men do.

Diagnosis and Treatment

The death rate from heart disease is falling faster for men than it is for women. This may be due in part to a lack of recognition and treatment of risk factors or symptoms of heart disease in women. Women are less likely to receive major diagnostic and therapeutic (treatment) procedures than men. Consider the following statistics from a review of over eighty thousand people hospitalized for heart disease in Maryland and Massachusetts (Ayanian and Epstein 1991):

- Men were 15 to 28 percent more likely than women to receive heart catheterization.

- Men were 27 to 45 percent more likely than women to receive balloon angioplasties and CABG surgeries.

Additionally, the standard tests used to diagnose heart disease may not be as reliable for women. For example, the traditional exercise stress test (EKG) and the thallium stress test are less precise in identifying heart disease in women. Part of the reason for this may be that women's breasts show up on the scans as a defect. Dr. Rita Redberg (cited in Hales 1997), from the University of California at San Francisco, suggests that a stress echocardiogram test may be a better indicator of heart disease in women. This test uses sound waves to create an image of the heart during exercise.

Women may also have more side effects associated with major treatments for heart disease. For instance, while women are about half as likely as men to receive heart bypass operations, they are more likely to have complications or to die after these surgeries. However, women who survive heart bypass operations recover as well as men do, and women who have surgery fare better than women in comparable situations who do not have the surgery.

Women are less likely to receive the clot-dissolving medications (thrombolytics) than men, and when they do receive them, they tend to have more complications. On the other hand, some studies have shown that a greater proportion of women are saved by thrombolytic treatments than men.

Why do these differences in treatment exist? It may be due to the fact that women tend to be older than men when they have heart problems. Disorders in older persons may not be viewed as seriously as those in younger persons. For example, there may be a greater sense of urgency in treating a man in his forties—who is perceived as having many responsibilities of family, job, and so on—than for a sixty-five- or seventy-year-old woman. Older persons are also more likely to have other health problems such as diabetes, high blood pressure, and kidney or respiratory problems. These difficulties make some procedures or treatments riskier.

It is also more difficult to perform some procedures, like bypass operations, on women than on men. Women's arteries tend to be smaller and more delicate than men's, making it more challenging to perform bypass procedures. New techniques have begun to improve outcomes for women, and surgeons are adapting to working with women's smaller blood vessels.

Overall, it has been hard to reach conclusions about the best way to diagnose and treat heart disease in women, because the numbers of women studied have been relatively small. Results of current and future research projects will be helpful. Until then, it may be best to assume that women may benefit from the same tests and treatments for heart disease as men. This is supported by results of recent studies that have reported that women seem to respond as well as men to a variety of medical treatments for heart disease. If you or a loved one have heart disease, be assertive and direct in asking your doctor about which tests and treatments may be beneficial for you.

Emotional and Social Risks

In general, the cardiac health of both women and men is adversely affected by stress. Regardless of your gender, difficulties with depression, anxiety, and negative personality styles, such as Type A behavior pattern, have been linked with greater risks for developing heart disease and poorer recovery from heart problems. When compared to men, women may show greater vulnerability to certain factors. Also, the established risk factors for men may not apply as well for women. Documented psychosocial risks for heart disease in women include chronic troubling emotions; stress of juggling multiple responsibilities of work and family; lack of social support (including divorce); low social class; low educational level; and personal losses (death of loved one, death of child). Read on to learn more.

Depression and Stress

More and more studies are showing how harmful chronic levels of depression are to your heart—for all people. However, this is more of a concern for women, because women are twice as likely as men to become depressed.

Although women's hormones offer protection against developing heart disease, they seem to do the opposite for depression. Rates of depression in females become higher than in males at adolescence and tend to remain this way throughout life. This has been shown for women in many different cultures and across differing populations. Reproductive hormones, like estrogen, appear to affect certain chemicals in the brain that are associated with moods in a way that can lead to depression. This puts women at risk not only for general depressive disorders, but also for disorders specific to women.

For instance, a majority of women experience some changes in mood related to the premenstrual phase (PMS). From 5 to 10 percent of women have regular, significant difficulties with depression occurring premenstrually that interfere with their ability to function on a daily basis. A majority of women (50 to 80 percent) have minor, short-lived depressive reactions after childbirth.

Contrary to popular belief, most women going through menopause do not have higher rates of depressive disorders. However, women at this time in their lives do tend to have struggles with personal or social issues. Changing life roles, children moving out of the home, divorce, and loss of family members or friends due to death all increase chances for depression and anxiety.

Women are also more likely than men to have a history of traumatic experiences, such as incest or molestation, rape, or domestic violence. All of these contribute to greater likelihood of depression.

One of the biggest strains in women's lives may come from juggling multiple roles and duties. In modern society, it is not unusual for women to be some or even all of the following:

- Wife
- Mother
- Daughter
- Caretaker of elderly or disabled parents or relatives
- Professional worker outside the home
- Homemaker
- Volunteer
- Community servant

A recent study of professional women by Dixon, Dixon, and Spinner (1991) showed that those women who had heart disease were more likely to report tension in juggling their career with commitments to their spouse, children, friends, and extended family. In attempts to engage in too many activities, women often spread themselves too thin. Especially if you are a perfectionist, you may come to experience guilt and be self-critical because you can't get everything done as well as you would like. Even the richest, most successful women seem to struggle with issues of balancing careers with family and home life, as reported in Elsa Walsh's 1996 book, *Divided Lives: The Public and Private Struggles of Three Accomplished Women.* For the majority of women, pressures of financial strain, unreliability of childcare, and worries about the safety of children at childcare settings worsen the situation. This may lead to even greater social strain, which has been associated with poorer emotional adjustment for women.

What's often lost in this frenzied balancing act is time for activities that give life a positive balance: relaxation, self-pampering, hobbies, socializing with friends, intimacy and companionship with your partner. When your balance becomes tipped toward a chronic state of feeling overwhelmed or guilty, the long-term effects may contribute to heart strain, in both an emotional and physical sense.

Men and women exhibit similar physical responses to stress (increase in blood pressure and levels of stress hormones) while at work. But when they come home from work, men's physical responses to stress diminish. Women's remain high and may even escalate more at home—perhaps because they are resuming their second or third job for the day as wife, mother, homemaker. This appears to support the old adage: "A woman's work is never done."

Feelings of guilt about not spending enough time with the family, or not doing your best job at work, often battle with guilt over the thought of cutting back on some responsibilities. Interestingly, women are vulnerable not only to stressful events that happen to themselves, but they appear more vulnerable than men to suffering distress when a loved one is stressed.

Attempts to juggle so many roles may leave you feeling chronically tired, with little energy, grouchy, and demoralized. This syndrome has at times been described as *vital exhaustion* and has been linked to greater risk of heart disease, especially heart attacks (Appels and Mulder 1989).

Wives seem to suffer more than husbands when marriages have difficulties. A recent study suggested that although both partners suffer equally in response to their own job stresses, women experienced more distress associated with marital strain than their husbands did (Barnett et al. 1995). On the brighter side, women seem to benefit more from good marriages than husbands do. Women who are unmarried, divorced, bereaved, or childless have greater risks of heart disease than married women.

Social Support

If you are socially isolated, lonely, or lack emotional support from friends or family, then you are at increased risk of heart disease, whether you are male or female. The strain from being a primary caretaker for children and often for aging or disabled parents or relatives takes an additional toll on women. Women are also more likely to be a single parent than men, and this greatly increases stress levels.

Educational Level and Job Strain

In general, women of low educational levels and with low-paying jobs are at greater risk for heart disease than women holding professional jobs. Women appear more vulnerable to heart disease if they are both divorced and employed without a college degree in jobs such as clerical positions. If you perceive yourself as having subordinate status and a relative lack of control in your work, this can lead to dissatisfaction with your job and higher distress levels. The effects of this are even worse if you do not have a partner to provide emotional support and social contact. In many cases, this situation may evolve in women who choose to focus on the roles of wife and mother and don't prepare themselves educationally for having a job in the future. They depend on their partner financially. If things go awry, however, due to divorce or death of a spouse, the resulting financial strain may force them into the work force, even though they feel unprepared for this. Because of a lack of education, they have to settle for jobs that may be unsatisfying and offer little pay. The sum total of this can lead to frustration over unmet expectations, as well as anger, resentment, loneliness, and dissatisfaction with life in general. Chronically experiencing such feelings, especially if they are suppressed, can lead to physical consequences, including heart disease.

Type A Behavior Pattern

In healthy women, some studies have shown that having Type A characteristics (such as time pressure, hard-driving nature, aggressiveness, and irritability) increases chances for having a first heart attack. However, other studies looking at what predicts death in women who have had a heart attack suggest that qualities opposite to the traditional Type A behaviors put women at greater risk. Rather than feeling time pressured and emotionally reactive to challenges, women were more likely to die after a heart attack if they reported feeling slowed down and with lower levels of emotional reactivity to challenges. This may reflect depression.

In women, the Type A behavior pattern may be expressed differently than in men. In general, this behavior pattern has been described as an ongoing struggle to achieve more and more in less and less time, often in spite of real or imagined obstacles. A man's struggle is typically to achieve success in work, physical strength, or control or power. Women's struggles or pressures may more often be related to relationships. As a woman, you may struggle to be perfect in caring for everyone else's needs—even if it means neglecting your own needs. A constant struggle involved in juggling duties of work and home life, or in always trying to meet other's needs without regard for your own, can lead to a sense of time pressure, impatience, and irritability. Maintaining this emotionally draining routine for long time periods contributes to fatigue, frustration, and stress. Again, when exposed to enduring stress levels and to the physical responses to stress (for example, increased blood pressure and release of stress hormones in the blood), you are more likely to suffer a heart attack or other form of heart disease.

Hostility is also manifested differently in men than women. Few women show outwardly hostile behavior on a regular basis. Women may be more likely to turn hostile feelings inward and harbor feelings of resentment and bitterness or become nervous, agitated, and depressed. Suppressing anger has been associated with greater likelihood of heart attacks in women, especially for those women employed in low-paying, clerical-type jobs. Other studies have not found negative effects for women associated with holding anger in. Being rigid in your style of expressing anger may do the most harm. If you tend to always hold anger in, or if you tend to always voice it explosively, then you may be placing yourself at greater risk for heart disease. If you are flexible in expressing anger—sometimes suppressing feelings, and sometimes expressing them openly—you may be in the best position for protecting your emotional and physical well-being.

If you meet your demands with a positive sense of achievement and enjoy the challenges of your life, then juggling multiple roles and anxieties will probably not affect you adversely. On the other hand, if you have harsh expectations and demands of perfectionism for yourself that you can never meet, then you may drive yourself to exhaustion in your attempts to manage your responsibilities. In this case, you are more likely to have low self-esteem and devalue and criticize yourself—which can truly be a heart-breaking situation.

The Role of Hormones and Heart Disease

Menopause represents the transition from the reproductive stage to the nonreproductive stage of a woman's life. It is not a disorder, but a natural part of a woman's development. The main physical changes occurring at this time include reduced functioning of the ovaries and, eventually, the end of menstrual periods. Ovulation also eventually stops (eggs are no longer released from the ovaries), and the ovaries produce less of the reproductive hormone estrogen. As estrogen levels drop, women often notice physical and emotional changes. These changes can begin several years before periods stop. The average age at the last menstrual period is fifty-one, but this varies widely. Some women go through menopause at a much younger age.

Even before menopause, some women might not produce enough estrogen, for a variety of reasons. For example, losing a great deal of weight from an eating disorder (such as anorexia nervosa) or engaging in excessive exercise can lead your body to produce less estrogen. This can cause monthly periods to stop. In addition, if you have your ovaries removed by surgery, your estrogen levels will drop suddenly instead of slowly declining, as is characteristic during menopause. This sudden loss of estrogen can cause severe symptoms of menopause.

Common effects of low estrogen include

- Menstrual periods become irregular and eventually stop. Periods can stop or become irregular for reasons other than menopause, so you should have a checkup by your gynecologist to be sure.

- Hot flushes, or hot flashes, are the most common symptom of menopause. About three-fourths of women going through menopause have them. They include a sudden hot feeling; blushing of the face, neck, and chest; and sweating, perhaps followed by chills. These usually last a few minutes and occur from a few to many times per day. They are more common at night and can interfere with your sleep. Hot flashes may come and go for several years.

- You'll notice changes having to do with your vaginal or urinary tract. Decreased estrogen leads to thinning and less moisture in vaginal tissues. This can cause pain during sexual activities and perhaps more frequent vaginal infections. Some women may feel a need to urinate more often.

- Emotional changes may include feeling moody, irritable, and having problems with concentration or memory. These may be a result of the physical symptoms of menopause, or of other factors, such as stress. For example, loss of sleep due to stress can lead you to feel irritable.

- Certain physical disorders become more likely. In addition to heart disease, women have a greater risk for osteoporosis (weakening or thinning of the bones, making fractures—especially of the wrist, hip and spine—more frequent). Though broken bones may not sound serious, there is a marked increase in death rates associated with bone fractures. Up to one in five persons with a hip fracture dies within six months of the break. Deaths occur due to the problems caused by lack of activity, which may lead to blood clots, stroke, heart attack, or pneumonia. Lack of estrogen may also increase risk for Alzheimer's disease.

Many of the symptoms associated with low estrogen levels can be controlled with hormone replacement therapy (HRT). After menopause, replacing the estrogen that has declined or disappeared may be good preventative medicine for you. Taking estrogen as prescribed by a doctor—either in pill or patch form—appears to lower risk of heart disease and osteoporosis, as well as relieve symptoms of hot flashes and vaginal dryness. Most studies have examined the effect of estrogens taken orally in pill form, so the protective effects of the patch are as yet not as firmly established. Several recent studies, including a recent study of nurses at Harvard, have suggested that taking hormones can reduce your risk of death from heart disease by as much as 50 percent. Keep in mind, however, that hormones do not protect women completely from heart disease. Even before menopause, having a number of other risk factors, such as smoking and high cholesterol levels, puts you at a greater risk for problems like heart attacks.

If you still have your uterus, then taking estrogen alone appears to increase your risk for developing uterine cancer (also known as endometrial cancer). Combining another hormone called progestin, or progesterone, with the estrogen can eliminate this risk. In fact, women taking both estrogen and progesterone have a lower risk of uterine cancer than women who take no hormones at all. If you've had a hysterectomy, then you needn't worry about uterine cancer, and taking estrogen alone appears to be safe.

Is Hormone Replacement Therapy Right for You?

While taking hormones can lower your risk for heart disease and osteoporosis and relieve symptoms such as hot flashes, vaginal dryness, and memory problems, like any treatment, hormone replacement is not free of risks. The decision to begin treatment depends on your medical history, symptoms, and risk of bone loss and of heart disease. Only you and your doctor can fully weigh the risks and benefits for you.

In general, the percentage of women taking hormone replacement appears relatively small. This may be due to a number of reasons, including a lack of information. Many women may not be aware of the risks associated with menopause. Utian and Schiff (1994) found that only about half of working women of menopausal ages were able to identify any long-term health worries associated with the years after menopause. Only 6 percent of those surveyed mentioned heart disease as a risk! Your doctor may be more likely to discuss the short-term side effects of hormone replacement with you than to give you information about the long-term health risks associated with menopause.

Even when women are informed of these risks, only about 20 percent of postmenopausal women are given prescriptions for hormone replacement. And less than half of those with prescriptions continue taking the hormones for more than a year. Sometimes hormone replacement therapy is avoided due to concerns about breast cancer. Though most studies do not support a strong link between hormone replacement and breast cancer, some indicate that a woman's chances of developing breast cancer are slightly increased by taking hormones for more than fifteen years. There is an estimated 1 to 2 percent increase in risk for breast cancer for each year of hormone replacement therapy. As recommended for other women, you should examine your breasts regularly and have physical exams and mammograms if you are taking hormones.

Hormone replacement therapy may also be avoided or discontinued due to side effects. About 10 percent of women taking hormones report troubling side effects. These may include breast tenderness, fluid retention or swelling, mood changes, or vaginal bleeding or spotting.

Unfortunately, there is confusion and misinformation about hormone replacement therapy after menopause. For example, a doctor recently publicly disagreed with the proven, long-term benefits of hormone replacement, and suggested, as an alternative, relying on estrogens that occur naturally in plant hormones. Tofu and other soy products and certain kinds of yams have substances similar to human estrogen and progesterone. For many health reasons, it is probably a good idea to eat foods like these that are rich in plant estrogens. However, most experts agree that this is not an adequate substitute for hormone replacement therapy. It probably can't supply enough estrogen to preserve your heart and bones as effectively as prescription hormones.

Although many women benefit from taking hormones, some may not be able to take them. If you've had breast or uterine cancer or liver disease, estrogen is not usually recommended. As with using any medication, the benefits must be weighed against the risks. Talk to your doctor and together decide if hormone replacement therapy may be right for you.

Protecting Your Heart

If you have traditional or nontraditional risk factors for heart disease, refer to the chapters in parts 3 and 4 for help in making lifestyle changes. If you've reached or passed menopause, talk to your family doctor or gynecologist about whether hormone replacement therapy may be beneficial for you in reducing risks of developing heart disease. In addition, consider the following options to help you successfully juggle your many responsibilities and provide protection for your heart:

- Maintain a balance in your life of positive, relaxing, self-nurturing activities to counter effects of the demanding stresses in your life.

- Try to maintain a positive outlook. View your responsibilities as challenges that can be enjoyable and of benefit to your life rather than as stresses that drain you. Appreciate all that you contribute to the many areas of your life instead of worrying about whether you are doing enough. Let go of guilt.

- Set aside time for yourself every day. Engaging in your favorite relaxing activities for as little as ten to thirty minutes per day can be of benefit. Ideas include stretching exercises, yoga, meditation, listening to your favorite kind of music, taking a warm bath, giving yourself a manicure or pedicure, reading for pleasure.

- Exercise regularly. Exercise is one of the best ways to reduce tension and stay fit emotionally as well as physically. It also helps improve sleep.

- Be flexible in the way you express feelings. Sometimes it's appropriate to withhold feelings and just let conflicts pass, and other times it's very important to assertively express your feelings.

- Learn to say "no" to avoid overextending yourself and to protect downtime for yourself.

- Hold a family meeting to discuss reorganizing your life and responsibilities. Delegate as many duties as possible and as is fair. If financially possible, hire outside help to assist with housework, baby-sitting, and yard work. If not, redistribute chores within your family. Doing this can free up your time to spend on activities that refresh and refuel you so you can be a more well-adjusted person for yourself and for all your loved ones.

- Regularly seek social support. Set regular one-on-one time with your husband or partner. Regularly spend time with friends.

- Keep a journal. Spend a few minutes each day, or at least every few days, writing about your feelings. Doing this is not only beneficial for your emotional well-being, but it can boost your immune system as well.

- If your attempts to improve your responses to stress in your life still leave you feeling depressed, anxious, or with marital difficulties, ask your doctor or family or friends for a referral to a mental health professional. Counseling has been shown to be effective in alleviating disorders like depression, and thereby can help you strengthen your heart as well.

You now have the tools you need to understand what your risks may be for developing heart disease and what you can do to protect your heart. It's now up to you to make the time to care for yourself. Good luck!

Epilogue

Before you opened this book, you were probably already familiar with the traditional risk factors for developing heart disease. You may even have heard about the less widely known, but no less dangerous, nontraditional risk factors.

However, you may have had difficulty accepting the notion that factors such as your emotions and personality style could actually be bad for your heart. We hope we've increased your awareness of how important thoughts and emotions are to your cardiac health. And if you're not yet convinced, we hope you will at least keep an open mind about heart therapy and experiment with suggestions to improve the way you deal with stress. You have nothing to lose in doing this and much to gain in strengthening both your heart and your mind. We wish you success in your efforts to protect and regain your heart health.

APPENDIX A

Glossary of Common Cardiac Terms

ACE (Angiotensin Converting Enzyme) Inhibitor: A class of drugs used to treat high high blood pressure and heart failure.

Acute myocardial infarction: Same as myocardial infarction, or heart attack. A portion of the heart muscle dies as a result of blockage of a narrowed coronary artery.

Adrenaline: A hormone produced in the body's fight-or-flight response; also called epinephrine.

Aerobic: Exercise that requires oxygen for energy production and can be sustained for long periods of time. Examples include walking, jogging, or swimming.

Anaerobic: Exercise that does not require oxygen for energy production and thus cannot be sustained for long periods of time. An example is weight lifting.

Angina: Discomfort and pain in the chest that usually lasts two to ten minutes. It is a warning sign of heart disease and is triggered by exertion or emotional stress. It can get worse in cold weather, after eating, or when angry or time pressured. Discomfort goes away with rest or by taking nitroglycerin.

Angiogram: An X ray of the heart or blood vessels after a dye is injected into the bloodstream.

Angioplasty: Also called percutaneous transluminal coronary angioplasty (PTCA); a technique in which a balloon is inflated in an artery of the heart that has become narrowed in order to dilate it.

Anticoagulant: A class of drugs that slows the clotting of blood, and helps prevent formation of new clots.

Antihypertensive: A class of drugs that lowers blood pressure.

Antilipids: Drugs that lower level of lipids (fats) in the blood.

Aorta: The largest artery in the body; it carries oxygenated blood from the left ventricle of the heart to its many branches in the rest of the body.

Arrhythmia: Irregular heartbeat, i.e., disturbance in the rhythm of the heart.

Arteries: Blood vessels that carry oxygenated blood away from the heart to the rest of the body.

Atherectomy: A procedure that widens a narrowed blood vessel by using an instrument to shave out the blockage; it is similar to angioplasty.

Atherosclerosis: A condition in which the walls of arteries become thick and irregular from a buildup of materials including cholesterol. When the deposits on a wall start to protude, the artery becomes narrowed and the flow of blood is obstructed. This can occur in any artery of the body.

Atria: The plural of the two upper chambers of the heart.

Atrial fibrillation: An irregular heartbeat that results from disturbances in the function of the atria.

Beta blocker: A class of drugs that slows heart rate, lowers blood pressure, and therefore is used to treat high blood pressure, angina, and other cardiac problems.

Calcium channel blocker: A class of drugs that blocks spasms of the artery; it is used to treat high blood pressure and angina.

Capillary: Tiny blood vessels that carry oxygen-rich blood to the tissues of the body.

Cardiac catheterization: A procedure in which a tube is inserted into an artery in the arm or leg and guided to the heart. A dye is then injected and X rays are taken of the coronary arteries, heart chambers, and valves.

Cardiovascular: Refers to the heart and blood vessels.

Cholesterol: A substance carried in the bloodstream that is both made in the body and found in many foods. When present in excess amounts, it sticks to artery walls, thereby causing narrowing of the artery.

Coronary arteries: Blood vessels that supply the heart itself with oxygen and nutrients.

Coronary artery bypass graft (CABG): A surgical procedure in which a graft is sewn around an area of blockage in a coronary artery, allowing blood to be detoured to the heart.

Coronary heart disease (CHD) or coronary artery disease (CAD): Disease of the arteries that supply the heart itself; the disease is primarily caused by the buildup of fatty deposits on the walls of the arteries.

Diastolic pressure: The measurement of the force of the blood against the artery walls when the heart is at rest.

Diuretic: Drug that removes excess fluids and salt from the body. It is used to treat high blood pressure.

Electrocardiogram (EKG or ECG): A device that records the electrical impulses of the heart; it is the first test performed to determine how the heart is functioning.

High-density lipoprotein (HDL): A carrier of cholesterol from arteries to the liver where cholesterol is then disposed; it is also referred to as the good, or healthy, cholesterol.

Holter monitor: An EKG recorded over a period of twenty-four hours while the person is conducting daily activities.

Hypertension: High blood pressure.

Ischemia: A condition in which not enough oxygen is supplied to the heart because of narrowed coronary arteries.

Lipid: A fatty substance that is insoluble in blood.

Lipoprotein: Combination of a lipid and protein that makes it possible for the lipid to travel in the bloodstream. Lipoproteins carry cholesterol.

Low-density lipoprotein (LDL): The main carrier of harmful cholesterol; it is often referred to as the bad cholesterol.

Myocardial infarction: Heart attack.

Nitroglycerin: A drug that is used to treat angina by causing the blood vessels to dilate.

Peripheral vascular disease: Narrowing of the blood vessels that carry blood to the legs.

Plaque: Hard fatty materials including deposits of cholesterol and other substances that become embedded in the artery wall and, with time, cause narrowing or blockage of the artery.

Saturated fat: A dietary fat (fat that is consumed through food consumption) that can result in coronary artery disease if too much is consumed, since foods that are high in saturated fat tend to be high in cholesterol as well.

Systolic pressure: The measurement of the force of the blood against the artery walls when the heart is contracting.

Tachycardia: An abnormally fast heartbeat at rest.

Thallium stress test: A test that involves taking images of the heart while the patient is exercising on a treadmill.

Thrombolytic: A drug that is used to break up existing clots and thus minimize heart damage; it is also known as clot-buster.

Triglyceride: One of the fats in the bloodstream.

Valve: A part of the heart that prevents backflow of blood between the heart chambers.

Vasodilator: A drug that dilates the blood vessels, allowing blood to flow more freely.

Ventricles: The two lower chambers of the heart.

Appendix B

Suggestions for Further Reading

Coronary Heart Disease/Heart Attack

Clayman, C. 1994. *The American Medical Association's Family Medical Guide.* New York: Random House.

Lorig, K., H. Holman, D. Sobel, D. Laurent, V. Gonzalez, and M. Minor. 1994. *Living a Healthy Life With Chronic Conditions: Self-Management of Heart Disease, Arthritis, Stroke, Diabetes, Asthma, Bronchitis, Emphysema, and Others.* Palo Alto, Calif.: Bull Publishing Company.

Mended Hearts: A nationwide patient support organization composed of people with heart disease, their families, medical professionals, and other interested persons. For more information about the Mended Hearts chapter in your area, contact your local American Heart Association office at (800) AHA-USA1. You can also call the Mended Hearts office in Dallas at (214) 706-1442 or visit their Web site at www.mendedhearts.org.

Nutrition (Healthy Diet)

DeBakey, M., A. M. Gotto, L. W. Scott, and J. P. Foreyt. 1986. *The Living Heart Diet.* New York: Simon and Schuster.

Personality

Daldrup, R., and D. Gust. 1990. *Freedom From Anger.* New York: Pocket Books.

Eliot, R. 1984. *Is It Worth Dying For?* New York: Bantam Books.

Friedman, M., and D. Ulmer. 1984. *Treating Type A Behavior and Your Heart.* New York: Ballantine Books.

Hankins, G., and C. Hankins. 1993. *Prescription for Anger: Coping With Angry Feelings and Angry People.* New York: Warner Books.

McKay, M., P. Rogers, and J. McKay. 1989. *When Anger Hurts.* Oakland, Calif.: New Harbinger Publications.

Sobel, D., and R. Ornstein. 1996. *The Healthy Mind, Healthy Body Handbook.* Los Altos, Calif.: DRx.

Williams, R., and V. Williams. 1993. *Anger Kills: Seventeen Strategies for Controlling the Hostility That Can Harm Your Health.* New York: Random House.

Stress, Anxiety, Communication Skills

Benson, H. 1974. *The Relaxation Response.* New York: Morrow.

Bolton, R. 1979. *People Skills.* New York: Simon and Schuster.

Bourne, E. J. 1990. *The Anxiety and Phobia Workbook,* second edition. Oakland, Calif.: New Harbinger Publications.

Davis, M., E. R. Eshelman, and M. McKay. 1995. *The Relaxation and Stress Reduction Workbook,* fourth edition. Oakland, Calif.: New Harbinger Publications.

Ellis, A. 1975. *A New Guide to Rational Living.* North Hollywood, Calif.: Wilshire Books.

Klein, A. 1989. *The Healing Power of Humor.* Los Angeles: Jeremy P. Tarcher.

Kushner, H. 1981. *When Bad Things Happen to Good People.* New York: Avon Books.

McKay, M., M. Davis, and P. Fanning. 1997. *Thoughts and Feelings: The Art of Cognitive Stress Intervention,* second edition. Oakland, Calif.: New Harbinger Publications.

Ornish, D. 1990. *Dr. Dean Ornish's Program for Reversing Heart Disease.* New York: Ballantine Books.

————. 1982. *Stress, Diet and Your Heart*. New York: Henry Holt and Co.

Siegel, B. 1986. *Love, Medicine and Miracles: Lessons Learned about Self-Healing from a Surgeon's Experience with Exceptional Pain*. New York: Harper and Row.

Quitting Smoking

Stevic-Rust, L., and A. Maximin. 1996. *The Stop Smoking Workbook*. Oakland, Calif.: New Harbinger Publications.

Women

American Heart Association. 1989. *The Silent Epidemic: The Truth About Women and Heart Disease*. Dallas: American Heart Association.

————. 1995. *Heart and Stroke Facts: 1995 Supplement*. Dallas: American Heart Association.

Fisher, R., and W. Ury. 1981. *Getting to Yes: Negotiating Agreement Without Giving In*. Boston: Houghton Mifflin.

Helfant, C. 1993. *The Women's Guide to Fighting Heart Disease*. New York: Berkley.

Pennebaker, J. 1990. *Opening Up: The Healing Power of Confiding In Others*. New York: William Morrow.

Schaef, A. 1990. *Meditations for Women Who Do Too Much*. San Francisco: HarperSanFrancisco.

Seligman, M. 1991. *Learned Optimism*. New York: Alfred A. Knopf.

Sobel, D., and R. Ornstein. 1996. *The Healthy Mind, Healthy Body Handbook*. Los Altos, Calif.: DRx.

The National Public Service Campaign on "The Difference in a Woman's Heart" offers materials to help women assess their risks for heart disease. You can call them at (800) 866-0400 for a copy of "Your Heart Health Record" to assess your risks for heart disease.

Sex and Relationships

Barbach, L. 1982. *For Each Other: Sharing Sexual Intimacy*. New York: Doubleday.

Chapunoff, E. 1991. *Sex and the Cardiac Patient*. Miami Beach, Fla: Bendy Books, Inc.

Godeck, G. 1993. *1001 Ways to Be Romantic.* Weymouth, Mass.: Casablanca Press.

Hendrix, H. 1988. *Getting the Love You Want: A Guide for Couples.* New York: Harper and Row.

Knopf, J., and M. Seiler. 1990. *Inhibited Sexual Desire.* New York: Warner Books.

Lerner, H. 1985. *The Dance Of Anger: A Woman's Guide to Changing the Patterns of Intimate Relationships.* New York: Harper and Row.

Renshaw, D. 1995. *Seven Weeks to Better Sex.* New York: Random House.

Sobel, D., and R. Ornstein. 1996. *The Healthy Mind, Healthy Body Handbook.* Los Altos, Calif.: DRx.

Zilbergeld, B. 1993. *The New Male Sexuality: The Truth About Men, Sex and Pleasure.* New York: Bantam Books.

Imagery Tapes

Fanning, B. 1992. *Visualization for Stress Reduction.* Oakland, Calif.: New Harbinger Publications.

Naparstek, B. 1993. *Heart Disease: Part of Health Journeys.* Los Angeles: Time Warner Audio Books. Call (800) 800-8661.

Sanders, H. 1995. *Peaceful Body, Quiet Mind.* Oakland, Calif.: New Harbinger Publications.

References

Aavedra, B. W. 1992 *Meditations for New Mothers*. New York: Workman Publishing.

Albert, C., B. McGovern, J. Newell, and J. Ruskin. 1996. Sex differences in cardiac arrest survivors. *Circulation* 93(6):1170-1176.

Allan, R., and S. Scheidt, editors. 1996. *Heart and Mind: The Practice of Cardiac Psychology*. Washington, D. C.: American Psychological Association.

American College of Cardiology/American Hospital Association. 1996. *Guidelines for the Management of Patients with Acute MI*.

American Heart Association. 1989. *The Silent Epidemic: The Truth About Women and Heart Disease*. Dallas: American Heart Association.

American Heart Association. 1995. *Heart and Stroke Facts*. Dallas: American Heart Association.

Anderson, K., P. Odell, P. Wilson, and W. Kannel. 1991. An updated coronary risk profile: A statement for health professionals. *Circulation*, 83:356-372.

Anderson, K., P. Odell, P. Wilson, and W. Kannel. 1993. Cardiovascular disease risk profiles. *American Heart Journal*, 121:293–298.

Appels, A., and P. Mulder. 1989. Fatigue and heart disease: The association between vital exhaustion and past, present, and future coronary heart disease. *Journal of Psychosomatic Research* 33:727–738.

Ayanian, J., and A. Epstein. 1991. Differences in use of procedures between men and women hospitalized for coronary heart disease. *New England Journal of Medicine* 325(4):221–225.

Ayanian, J., E. Guadagnoli, and P. Cleary. 1995. Physical and psychosocial functioning of women and men after coronary artery bypass surgery. *Journal of American Medical Association* 274(22): 1767–1770.

Barbach, L. 1982. *For Each Other: Sharing Sexual Intimacy.* New York: Doubleday.

Barefoot, J., and M. Schroll. 1996. Symptoms of depression, acute myocardial infarction and and total mortality in a community sample. *Circulation* 93:1976–1980.

Barnett, R., S. Raudenbush, R. Brennan, J. Pleck, and N. Marshall. 1995. Change in job and marital experiences and change in psychological distress: a longitudinal study of dual-career couples. *Journal of Personality and Social Psychology* 69(5):839–850.

Baron-Faust, R. 1995. *Preventing Heart Disease: What Every Woman Should Know.* San Francisco: Hearst Books.

Becker, L., C. Pepine, R. Bonsall. et al. 1996. Left ventricular, peripheral vascular, and neurobehavioral responses to mental stress in normal middle aged men and women. Reference group for the Psychophysiological Investigations of Myocardial Ischemia (PIMI) study. *Circulation* 94(11):2768–2777.

Benson, H. 1974. *The Relaxation Response.* New York: Morrow.

Bertolet, B., and J. Hill. 1989. Unrecognized Myocardial Infarction. In *Acute Myocardial Infarction,* edited by C. Pepine. Philadelphia: F.A. Davis Company.

Bohlen, J., J. Held, M. Wanderson, and R. Patterson. 1984. Heart rate pressure production and oxygen uptake during psychosexual activities. *Archives of Internal Medicine* 144:1745–48.

Brezinka, V., and F. Kittel. 1996. Psychosocial factors of coronary heart disease in women: A review. *Social Science and Medicine* 42(10): 1351–1365.

Budhoff, M., D. Georgiou, and A. Brody. 1996. Ultrafast computed tomography as a diagnostic modality in the detection of CAD: A multicenter study. *Circulation* 93(5):898–904.

Casscells, S. 1996. UT-Houston implements gender-based screening for heart disease. *UT-Houston Online Newspaper* February.

Chapunoff, E. 1991. *Sex and the Cardiac Patient.* Miami Beach, Fla: Bendy Books, Inc.

Chesney, M. 1992. Social isolation, depression and heart disease: Research on women broadens the agenda. *Psychosomatic Medicine* 55:434–435.

Clay, R. 1997. Laughter offers subtle and not so subtle boosts to health. *American Psychiatric Association Monitor* 28(9).

Clayman, C. 1994. *The American Medical Association's Family Medical Guide.* New York: Random House.

Cohen, S., and T. A. Wills. 1985. Stress, social support and the buffering hypothesis. *Psychological Bulletin.* 98(2):310–357

Condos, W. 1996. You can have a heart attack without knowing it. Lake Charles: Cardiovascular Institute of the South. www.cardio.com\articles\silent.HTM.

Consumer Guide. 1989. *Cholesterol: Your Guide for a Healthy Heart.* Publications International: Lincolnwood, Ill.

Consumer Reports. 1992. Are you eating right? *Consumer Reports,* 644–655.

Cunningham, M., T. Lee, E. Cook, D. Brand, G. Rouan, M. Weisberg, and L. Goldman. 1989. The effect of gender on the probability of myocardial infarction among emergency department patients with acute chest pain: A report from the Multicenter Chest Pain Study Group. *Jounal of General Internal Medicine,* 4(5):392–398.

Daldrup, R., and D. Gust. 1990. *Freedom From Anger.* New York: Pocket Books.

DeBusk, R. 1996. Sexual activity triggering myocardial infarction: One less thing to worry about. *Journal of American Medical Association* 275(18):1447–1448.

Denollet, J., S. Sys, N. Stroobant, H. Rombouts, T. Gillebert, and D. Brutsaert. 1996. Personality as independent predictor of long-term mortality in patients with coronary heart disease. *Lancet* 347:417–421.

DSM-IV. 1994. Diagnostic and Statistical Manual of Mental Disorders, fourth edition. Washington, D. C.: American Psychiatric Association.

Dixon, J., J. Dixon, and J. Spinner. 1991. Tensions between career and interpersonal commitments as a risk factor for cardiovascular disease among women. *Women and Health* 17:33–57.

Dunbar, F. 1943. *Psychosomatic Diagnosis.* New York: Paul B. Hoeben, Inc.

Eaker, E., J. Pinsky, and W. Castelli. 1992 Myocardial infarction and coronary death among women: Psychosocial predictors from a twenty year follow-up of women in the Framingham study. *American Journal of Epidemiology* 135:854–64.

Eliot, R., and D. Breo. 1984. *Is It Worth Dying For?* New York: Bantam Books.

Ellis, A. 1975. *A New Guide to Rational Living.* North Hollywood, Calif.: Wilshire Books.

Ellis, S., W. Weintraub, D. Holmes, R. Shaw, D. Block, and S. King. 1997. Relation of operator volume and experience to procedural outcome of percutaneous coronary revascularization at hospitals with high interventional volumes. *Circulation* 95(11):2479–2484.

Engebretson, T., and C. Stoney. 1995. Anger expression and lipid concentrations. *International Journal of Behavioral Medicine* 2(4): 281–298.

Everson, S. A., D. E. Goldberg, et al. 1996. Hopelessness and risk of mortality and incidence of myocardial infarction and cancer. *Psychosomatic Medicine* 58, 2:113–121.

Fawcett, J. 1992. Suicide risk factors in depressive disorders and in panic disorders. *Journal of Clinical Psychiatry*, 53:9–13.

Fawcett, J., D. C. Clark, and K. A. Busch. 1993. Assessing and treating the patient at risk for suicide. *Psychiatric Annals* 23:244–255.

Feiden, M. 1989. *The Calorie Factor: The Dieter's Companion.* Simon & Schuster.

Feighner, J. P., E. A. Gardner, J. A. Johnston, S. R. Batey, M. A. Khayrallah, J. A. Archer, and C. G. Lineberry. 1991. Double-blind comparison of bupropion and fluoxetine in depressed outpatients. *Journal of Clinical Psychiatry* 52:329–335.

Fetters, J., E. Peterson, L. Shaw, L. Newby, and R. Califf. 1996. Sex-specific differences in coronary artery disease risk factors, evaluation, and treatment: Have they been adequately evaluated? *American Heart Journal* 131(4):796–813.

Fisher, R., and W. Ury. 1981. *Getting to Yes: Negotiating Agreement Without Giving In.* Boston: Houghton Mifflin.

Frasure-Smith, N. 1991. In-hospital symptoms of psychological stress as predictors of long-term outcome after acute myocardial infarction in men. *The American Journal of Cardiology* 67:121–27.

Frasure-Smith, N., F. Lesperance, and M. Talajic. 1993. Depression following myocardial infarction: Impact on six month survival. *Journal of American Medical Association* 270:1819–1825.

———. 1995. The impact of negative emotions on prognosis following myocardial infarction: Is it more than depression? *Health Psychology*14(5):388–98.

Freedland, K., R. Carney, R. Krone, et al. 1991. Psychological factors in silent myocardial ischemia. *Psychosomatic Medicine* 53:13–24.

Friedman, H., editor. 1992. *Hostility, Coping and Health.* Washington, DC.: American Psychological Association.

Friedman, M., N. Fleischmann, and V. Price. 1996. Diagnosis of Type A behavior pattern. In *Heart and Mind: The Practice of Cardiac*

Psychology, edited by R. Allan, and S. Scheidt. Washington, D. C.: American Psychological Association.

Friedman, M., and G. Ghandour. 1993. Medical diagnosis of Type A behavior. *American Heart Journal* 126:607–618.

Friedman, M., and R. H. Rosenman. 1974 *Type A Behavior and Your Heart.* New York: Alfred A. Knopf.

Friedman, M., and D. Ulmer. 1984. *Treating Type A Behavior and Your Heart.* New York: Ballantine Books.

Fry, H. 1997. Humor and its healing effects. *APA Monitor* 27(9).

Gill, J. S., A. Z. Zezulka, and M. J. Shipley. 1986. Stroke and alcohol consumption. *New England Journal of Medicine* 315:1041–46.

Godeck, G. 1993. *1001 Ways to Be Romantic.* Weymouth, Mass.: Casablanca Press.

Goodman, M., J. Quigley, G. Moran, H. Meilman, and M. Sherman. 1996. Hostility predicts restenosis after percutaneous transluminal angioplasty. *Mayo Clinic Proceedings* 71:729–734.

Guzzetta, C. 1989. Effects of relaxation and music therapy on patients in a coronary care unit with presumptive acute myocardial infarction. *Heart and Lung* 18(6):609–616.

Hafen, B., K. Frandsaen, K. Karren, and K. Hooker. 1992. *The Health Effects of Attitudes, Emotions, and Relationships.* Provo, UT: EMS Associates.

Hales, D. 1997. Women's health enemy number one. *Ladies Home Journal* April, 110–116.

Hammond, C. 1997. Management of menopause. *American Family Physician* 55(5):1667–1674.

Hankins, G., and C. Hankins. 1993. *Prescription for Anger: Coping with Angry Feelings and Angry People.* New York: Warner Books.

Helfant, R. 1993. *The Women's Guide to Fighting Heart Disease.* New York: Berkley.

Helmers, K., D. Posluszny, and D. Krantz. 1994. Associations of hostility and coronary artery disease: A review of studies. In *Anger, Hostility and the Heart,* edited by A. W. Siegman and T. W. Smith Hillsdale, N. J.: Erlbaum.

Hennekens, C., M. Dyken, and V. Fuster. 1997. Aspirin as a therapeutic agent in cardiovascular disease: A statement for healthcare professionals from the American Heart Association. *Circulation* 96(8):2751–2753.

House, J. S. 1981. *Work Stress and Social Support.* Reading, Mass.: Addison-Wesley.

Jacobs, S., and J. Sherwood. 1996. The cardiac psychology of women and heart disease. In *Heart and Mind*, edited by R. Allan and S. Scheidt. Washington, D. C.: American Psychiatric Association.

Jacobson, E. 1974. *Progressive Relaxation*. Midway reprint. Chicago: The University of Chicago Press.

Jiang, W., M. Babyak, D. Krantz, R. Waugh. et al. 1996. Mental stress induced myocardial ischemia and cardiac events. *Journal of the American Medical Association* 275(21):1651–1656.

Jorgensen, R. S., B. T. Johnson, M. E. Kolodziej, and S. C. Schreer. 1996. Elevated blood pressure and personality: A meta-analytic review. *Psychological Bulletin* 120:293–320.

Joseph, A. M. 1996. Nicotine replacement treatment for cardiac patients. *American Journal of Health Behavior* 20(5), 261-269.

Kendrick, J., and R. Merritt. 1996. Women and smoking: an update for the 1990s. *American Journal of Obstetrics and Gynecology* 175: 528–535.

Kannel, W. 1986. Silent myocardial ischemia and infarction: insights from the Framingham study. *Cardiology Clinics* 4(4):583–591.

Kenyon, L. 1995. Can sexual intimacy survive serious illness? *St. Joseph Mercy Hospital Health Tips* Summer:6.

Kenyon, L., and M. Ketterer. 1991. Level of somatic awareness and ain perception in patients with acute myocardial infarction. *Proceedings of the Society of Behavioral Medicine*, XII, 83 (Abstract).

Kenyon, L., M. Ketterer, M. Gheorghiade, and S. Goldstein. 1991. Psychological factors related to prehospital delay in acute myocardial infarction. *Circulation* 84:1969–1976.

Kenyon, L., M. Ketterer, and R. Preisman. 1991. Psychological factors relevant to the prehospital and inhospital phases of acute myocardial infarction. *Henry Ford Medical Journal* 39:176–183.

Ketterer, M. 1993. Secondary prevention of ischemic heart disease: The case for aggressive behavioral monitoring and intervention. *Psychosomatics* 34:478–484.

Ketterer, M., J. Brymer, K. Rhoads, P. Kraft, and L. Kenyon. 1994. Snoring and the severity of coronary artery disease in men. *Psychosomatic Medicine* 56:232–236.

Ketterer, M., L. Kenyon, B. Foley, J. Brymer, K. Rhoads, P. Kraft, and W. Lovallo. 1996. Denial of depression as an independent correlate of coronary artery disease. *Journal of Health Psychology* 1(1):93–105.

Ketterer, M., L. Kenyon, and M. Gheorghiade. 1994. A randomly assigned, controlled pilot study of triaging and psychiatric consultation in acute myocardial infarction. *Psychosomatic Medicine* 53:173 (Abstract).

Ketterer, M., L. Kenyon, K. Rhoades, J. Brymer, and W. Lovallo. 1991. Alexithymia and CAD status in males undergoing coronary angiography. *Psychosomatic Medicine* 53:227–228.

Ketterer, M., L. Kenyon, K. Rhoades, J. Brymer, and W. LoVallo. 1991. Indices of depression and ischemic heart disease. *Proceedings of the Academy of Psychosomatic Medicine* 39:58.

Ketterer, M., J. Brymer, K. Rhoads, P. Kraft, L. Kenyon, B. Foley, W. Lovallo, and C. Voight. 1996. Emotional distress among males with "syndrome X." *Journal of Behavioral Medicine* 19(5):455–467.

Kirschenbaum, D. S. 1994. *Weight Loss Through Persistence: Making Science Work For You*. Oakland, Calif.: New Harbinger Publications.

Knopf, J., and M. Seiler. 1990. *Inhibited Sexual Desire*. New York: Warner Books.

Kushi, L., A. Folsom, R. Prineas, P. Mink, Y. Wu, and R. Bostick. 1996. Dietary anitioxidants, vitamins and death from coronary heart disease in post menopausal women. *New England Journal of Medicine* 334(18):1156–1162.

Kusinitz, I., M. Fine, and editors of Consumer Reports Books. 1983. *Physical Fitness for Practically Everybody: The Consumer Union Report on Exercise*. Mount Vernon, New York: Consumers Union.

Lai, J., and W. Linden. 1992. Gender, age, expression style, and opportunity for anger release determines cardiovascular reaction to and recovery from anger provocation. *Psychosomatic Medicine* 54:297–310.

Latella, F. S., W. Conkling, and editors of Consumer Reports Books. 1989 *Get in Shape, Stay in Shape*. New York: Consumer Reports Books.

Lefcourt, H. M., K. Davidson, R. Shepherd, and M. Phillips. 1995. Perspective taking humor: Accounting for stress moderation, *Journal of Social and Clinical Psychology* 14(4):373–391.

Lesperance, F., N. Frasure-Smith, and M. Talajic. Major depression before and after myocardial infarction: its nature and consequences. *Psychosomatic Medicine* 58:99–109.

Linden, W., C. Stossel, and J. Maurice. 1996. Psychosocial intervention for patients with coronary artery disease: A meta-analysis. *Archives of Internal Medicine* 156:745–752.

Lorig, K., H. Holman, D. Sobel, D. Laurent, V. Gonzalez, and M. Minor. 1994. *Living a Healthy Life with Chronic Conditions: Self-Management of Heart Disease, Arthritis, Stroke, Diabetes, Asthma,*

Bronchitis, Emphysema and Others. Palo Alto, Calif.: Bull Publishing Company.

Maclure, M., J. Sherwood, M. Mittleman, et al. 1991. Increased risk of myocardial infarction onset within the 2 hours after awakening. (Abst.). *Circulation* 82:supplement I118.

Margolis, S., editor. 1996. Stress: How big a heart attack risk? *The Johns Hopkins Medical Newsletter: Health After 50* December, 1996, 8(10):1–2.

———. 1997. Bypassing bypass difficulties. *The Johns Hopkins Medical Letter: Health After 50* August, 9(6):1–2.

———. 1997. A consumer's guide to reproductive hormones. *The Johns Hopkins Medical Letter: Health After 50* September, 9(7):9(5)4–5.

———. 1997. Heart disease: The mind-body connection. *The Johns Hopkins Medical Letter: Health After 50* July, 9(5):4–5.

———. 1997. A new, better heart disease test. *The Johns Hopkins Medical Letter: Health After 50* June, 9(4):1–2.

Markovitz, J. H., K. A. Matthews, et al. 1996. Effects of hostility on platelet reactivity to psychological stress in coronary heart disease patients and in healthy controls. *Psychosomatic Medicine* 58: 143–149.

Matthews, K., S. Shumaker, D. Bowen, et al. 1997. Women's health initiative. *American Psychologist* 52(2):101–116.

Matthews, K., J. Siegel, K. Keiller, and M. Thompson. 1983. Determinants of decision to seek medical treatment by patients with acute myocardial infarction symptoms. *Journal of Personality and Social Psychology* 44:1144–56.

McKay, M., Rogers, P., McKay, J. 1989. *When Anger Hurts.* Oakland, Calif.: New Harbinger Publications.

Miller, S. 1987. Monitoring and blunting: Validation of a questionnaire to assess Different styles of coping with stress. *Journal of Personality and Social Psychology* 52:345–53.

Mittleman, M., M. Maclure, J. Sherwood. et al. 1995. Triggering of acute myocardial infarction onset by episodes of anger. *Circulation* 92:1720–25.

Mittleman, M., M. Maclure, G. Tofler, et al. 1993. Triggering of acute myocardial infarction by heavy physical exertion: Protect against triggering by regular exercise. *New England Journal of Medicine* 329:1677–1683.

Moen, E., C. Asher, D. Miller, W. Weaver, H. White, R. Califf, and E. Topol. 1997. Long-term follow-up of gender specific outcomes after thrombolytic therapy for acute myocardial infarction for the GUSTO-1 trial: Global utilization of streptokinase and tissue plasminogen activator for occluded coronary arteries. *Journal of Women's Health* 6(3):285–293.

Montgomery, S. A. 1993. Venlafaxine: A new dimension in antidepressant pharmacotherapy. *Journal of Clinical Psychiatry* 54:119–126.

Muller, J., M. Mittleman, M. Maclure, J. Sherwood, and G. Tofler. 1996. Triggering myocardial infarction by sexual activity: Low absolute risk and prevention by regular exercise. *Journal of American Medical Association* 275(18):1405–1409.

Muller, J., G. Tofler, and P. Stove. 1989. Circadian variation and triggers of onset of acute cardiovascular disease. *Circulation* 79: 733–744.

National Cholesterol Education Panel. 1988. *Archives of Internal Medicine* 148:36.

Netzer, C. T. 1991. *The Complete Book of Food Counts,* second edition. New York: Dell Publishing.

Nunes, E., K. Frank, and D. Kornfeld. 1987. Psychological treatment for Type A behavior pattern and for coronary heart disease: A meta-analysis of the literature. *Psychosomatic Medicine* 48:159–173.

Oldenburg, B., R. Perkins, and G. Andrews. 1985. Controlled trial of psychological intervention in myocardial infarction. *Journal of Consulting and Clinical Psychology* 53:852–859.

Ornish, D., S. Brown, L. Scherwitz, J. Billings, W. Armstrong, T. Ports. et al. 1990. Can lifestyle changes reverse coronary artery disease? *Lancet,* 336:129–133.

Pennebaker, J. 1990. *Opening Up: The Healing Power of Confiding in Others.* New York: William Morrow.

Petrie, K., D. Buick, and J. Weinman. 1996. Positive effects of illness reported by myocardial and breast cancer patients. Abstract. *Psychosomatic Medicine,* 58:76

Powell, L., L. Shaker, B. Jones. et al. 1993. Psychosocial predictors of mortality in 83 women with premature acute myocardial infarction. *Psychosomatic Medicine* 55:426–433.

Price, D. 1995. The heart of the matter: Too many women believe cardiovascular diseases are limited to men. *The Detroit News,* 2 October.

Price, V., M. Friedman, G. Ghandour, and N. Fleischmann. 1995. Relationship between insecurity and Type A behavior. *American Heart Journal* 129:488–91.

Rand, G. H. 1991. Choosing an antidepressant to treat depression. *American Family Physician* 43(3):847–854.

Renshaw, D. 1995. *Seven Weeks to Better Sex.* New York: Random House.

Rippe, J. M. and P. Amend. 1992. *The Exercise Exchange Program.* New York: Simon and Schuster.

Ryan, T., J. Anderson, E. Antinan, and B. Braniff. 1996. ACC/AHA guidelines for the management of patients with acute myocardial infarction. Report of the American College of Cardiology/American Heart Association Task Force on Practice Guidelines. *Circulation* 94:2341–2350.

Satir, V. 1972. *People Making.* Palo Alto, Calif.: Science and Behavior Books.

Schaef, A. 1990. *Meditations for Women Who Do Too Much.* San Fransisco: HarperSanFrancisco.

Scheier, M. F., et al. 1989. Dispositional optimism and recovery from coronary artery bypass surgery: The beneficial effects on physical and psychological well-being. *Journal of Personality and Social Psychology* 57:1024–1040.

Schover, L. and Jensen, S. 1988. *Sexuality and Chronic Illness: A Comprehensive Approach.* New York: Guilford Press.

Seligman, M. 1991. *Learned Optimism,* 2nd edition. New York: Alfred A. Knopf.

Siegel, W., D. Mark, N. Hlatky, et al. 1989. Exercise-induced silent ischemia: Effect of Type A behavior pattern on frequency and prognosis. *American Journal of Cardiology* 64:1280–83.

Shapiro, S., D. Sloan, L. Rosenberg, D. Kaufman, P. Stolley, and O. Miettinen. 1979. Oral contraceptive use in relation to myocardial infarction. *Lancet* 1:743–747.

Shaw, L., D. Miller, J. Romeis, D. Karge, L. Younis, and B. Chaitman. 1994. Gender differences in the noninvasive evaluation and management of patients with suspected coronary artery disease. *Annals of Internal Medicine* 120(7):559–566.

Smith, T. 1992. Hostility and health: Current status of a psychosomatic hypothesis. *Health Psychology* 11:139–150.

Sobel, D., and R. Ornstein. 1996. *The Healthy Mind, Healthy Body Handbook.* Los Altos, Calif.: DRx.

Sobel, D., and R. Ornstein. editors. 1996. Healthy anger: Let it out or keep it in? *Mind/Body Health* 2:1.

———. 1996. hostility, depression and heart disease. *Mind/Body Health* 3:1

———. 1996. Rx: Preparing for surgery, *Mind/Body Health* 5(2):3–6.

————. 1996. Sexual activity and heart attack: Not to worry. *Mind-Body Health* 5(1):1–2.

Speroff, L., P. Collins, D. Mishell, M. Stampfer, and J. Sullivan. 1997. Postmenopausal hormone therapy and the cardiovascular system. *Supplement: Contemporary OB/GYN* June, 4–32.

Stoney, C., and T. Engebretson. 1994. Anger and hostility: Potential mediators of the gender differences in coronary heart disease. In *Anger, Hostility and the Heart,* edited by A. W. Siegman. Hillsdale, N. J.: Erlbaum.

Stampfer, M.J., Colditz, G.A., Willett, W.C. 1988. A prospective study of moderate alcohol consumption and the risk of coronary disease and stroke in women. *New England Journal of Medicine* 319:267–273.

Stoney, C., K. Matthews, R. McDonald, and C. Johnson. 1988. Sex differences in lipoprotein, cardiovascular, and neuroendocrine responses to acute stress. *Psychophysiology* 25:645–656.

Tardif, G. 1989. Sexual activity after a myocardial infarction. *Archives of Physical Medicine and Rehabilitation* 70:763–66.

Tans, M., D. Jacobs, Y. Stern, et al. 1997. Effect of estrogen during menopause on risk and age at onset of Alzheimer's disease. *Lancet* 348:429–432.

Theisen, M., S. MacNeil, M. Lumley, M., Ketterer. et al. 1995. Psychosocial factors related to unrecognized acute myocardial infarction. *American Journal of Cardiology* 75:1211–13.

Thoresen, C., and L. Powell. 1992. Type A behavior pattern: New perspectives on theory, assessment and intervention. *Journal of Consulting and Clinical Psychology* 60:595–604.

Ting, H., T. Lee, J. Soukup, E. Cook, A. Tosteson, D. Brand, G. Rouan, and L. Goldman. 1991. Impact of physician experience on triage of emergency room patients with acute chest pain at three teaching hospitals. *American Journal of Medicine* 91(4):401–408.

Tofler, G., J. Muller, P. Stone. et al. 1992. Modifiers of timing and possible triggers of onset of acute myocardial infarction in the TIMI II population *Journal of the American College of Cardiology* 20:1045–55.

Tofler, G., P. Stone, M. Maclure. et al. 1990. Analysis of possible triggers of acute myocardial infarction (the MILIS study). *American Journal of Cardiology,* 66:22–27.

Uchino, B. and L. Cacioppo. 1996. The relationship between social support and physiological processes: A review with emphasis on underlying mechanisms and implications for health. *Psychological Bulletin* 119:488–531.

U.S. Department of Agriculture and U.S. Department of Health and Human Services. Nutrition and your health: Dietary guidelines for Americans, third edition. *Home and Garden Bulletin No. 232.* Washington D. C.: Government Printing Office.

Utian, W., and I. Schiff. 1994. Gallup survey on women's knowledge, information sources, and attitudes toward menopause and hormone replacement therapy. *Menopause* 1:39–48.

Walsh, E. 1996. *Divided Lives: The Public and Private Struggles of Three Accomplished Women.* New York: Anchor Books, Doubleday.

Wenger, N., L. Speroff, and B. Packard, editors. 1993. *Cardiovascular Health and Disease in Women.* Greenwich, Conn.: Le Jacq Communications.

White, J. 1992. Music therapy: an intervention to reduce anxiety in the myocardial infarction patient. *Clinical Nurse Specialist* 6(2): 58–63.

Whitehouse, W., D. Dinges, E. Orne, S. Keller. et al. 1996. Psychosocial and immune effects of self-hypnosis training for stress management throughout the first semester of medical school. *Psychosomatic Medicine* 58(3):249–263

Wild, R., E. Taylor, and A. Duchans. 1995. The gynecologist and the prevention of cardiovascular disease. *American Journal of Obstetrics and Gynecology* 172:1–13.

Williams, R., and V. Williams. 1993. *Anger Kills: Seventeen Strategies for Controlling the Hostility That Can Harm Your Health.* New York: Random House.

Williams, W. 1988. *Rekindling Desire: Bringing Your Sexual Relationship Back to Life.* Oakland, Calif.: New Harbinger Publications.

Zilbergeld, B. 1993. *The New Male Sexuality: The Truth About Men, Sex and Pleasure.* New York: Bantam Books.

Index

More New Harbinger Titles

LIVING WITH ANGINA
Explains the latest medical facts and shows what to do to reduce the risk of a heart attack and help you live life to the full.
Item HART Paperback $12.95

THE DAILY RELAXER
Presents the most effective and popular techniques for learning how to relax—simple, tension-relieving exercises that you can learn in five minutes and practice with positive results right away.
Item DALY Paperback, $12.95

THE HEADACHE AND NECK PAIN WORKBOOK
Combines the latest research with proven alternative therapies to help sufferers of head and neck pain understand and master their condition.   *Item NECK Paperback $14.95*

THE CHRONIC PAIN CONTROL WORKBOOK
A team of specialists in all areas of pain management detail the treatment strategies for managing and recovering from chronic pain.   *Item PN2 Paperback $17.95*

FIBROMYALGIA & CHRONIC MYOFASCIAL PAIN SYNDROME
This survival manual is the first comprehensive patient guide for managing these conditions. Readers learn how to identify trigger points, cope with chronic pain and sleep problems, and deal with the numbing effects of "fibrofog."   *Item FMS Paperback, $19.95*

PREPARING FOR SURGERY
Details tested techniques to prepare the mind and body for surgery—techniques that have been found to help decrease the need for postoperative pain medicine, reduce complications, and promote a quicker return to health.   *Item PREP Paperback, $17.95*

Call **toll-free 1-800-748-6273** to order. Have your Visa or Mastercard number ready. Or send a check for the titles you want to New Harbinger Publications, 5674 Shattuck Avenue, Oakland, CA 94609. Include $3.80 for the first book and 75¢ for each additional book to cover shipping and handling. (California residents please include appropriate sales tax.) Allow four to six weeks for delivery.

Prices subject to change without notice.

Some Other New Harbinger Self-Help Titles